the DIY Apothecary

CREATE YOUR OWN NATURAL BATH & BODY PRODUCTS

SUSAN R. BREWIN

FriesenPress
Suite 300 - 990 Fort St
Victoria, BC, V8V 3K2
Canada

www.friesenpress.com

First Edition — 2020

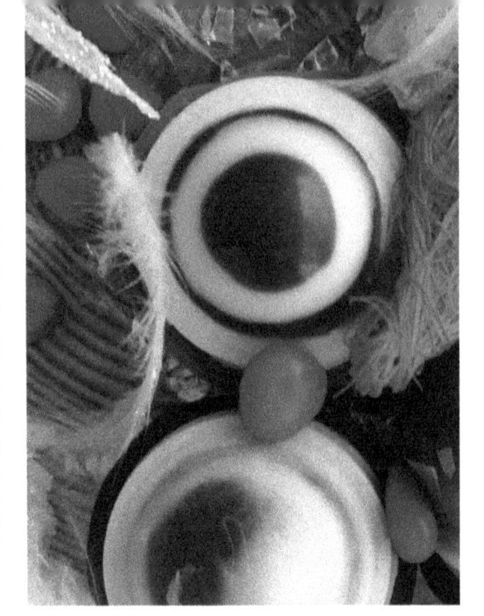

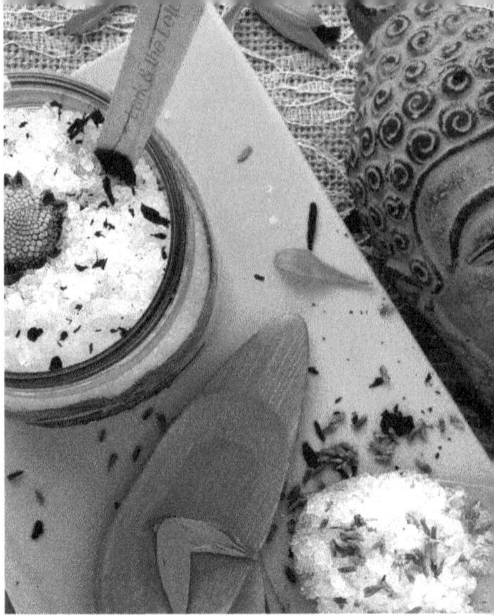

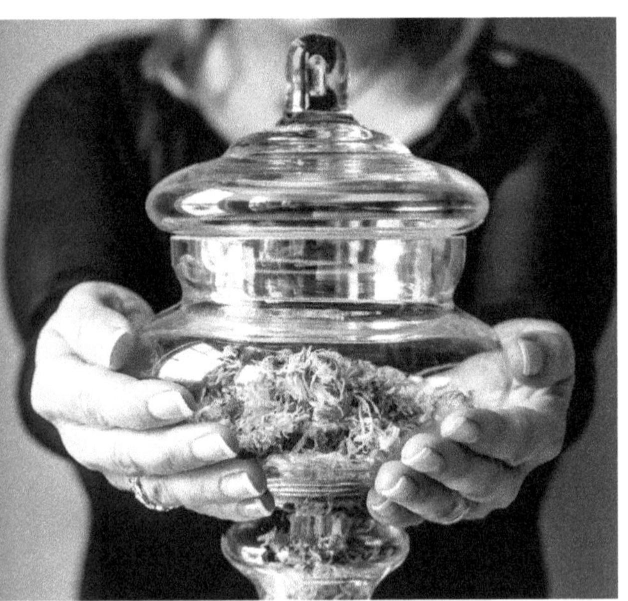

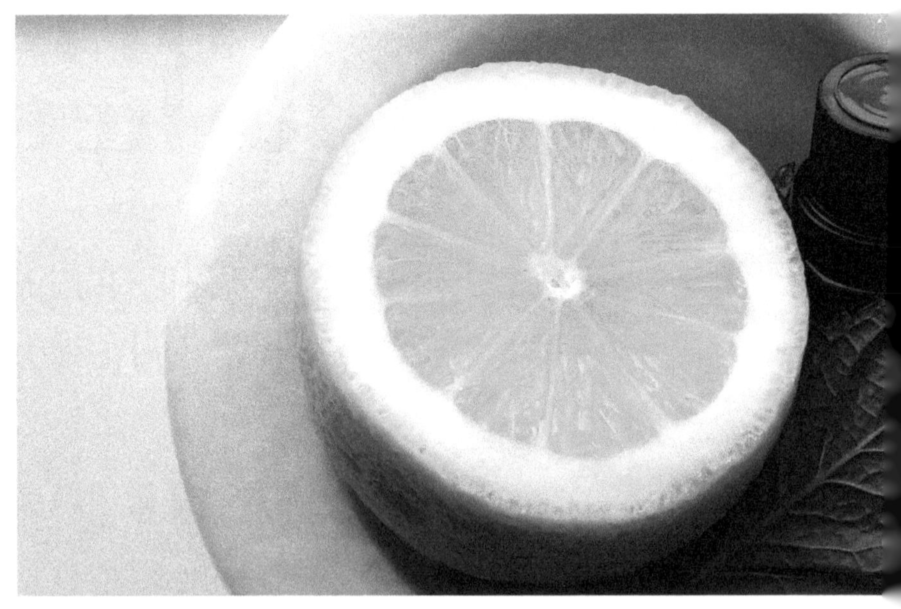

Photo Credits - images of author by Nat Caron
Images of products by Susan Brewin
Photography
Stock images by Pixabay.com

ISBN
978-1-5255-5889-4 (Hardcover)
978-1-5255-5890-0 (Paperback)
978-1-5255-5891-7 (eBook)
Health & Fitness, Aromatherapy

Distributed to the trade by
The Ingram Book Company

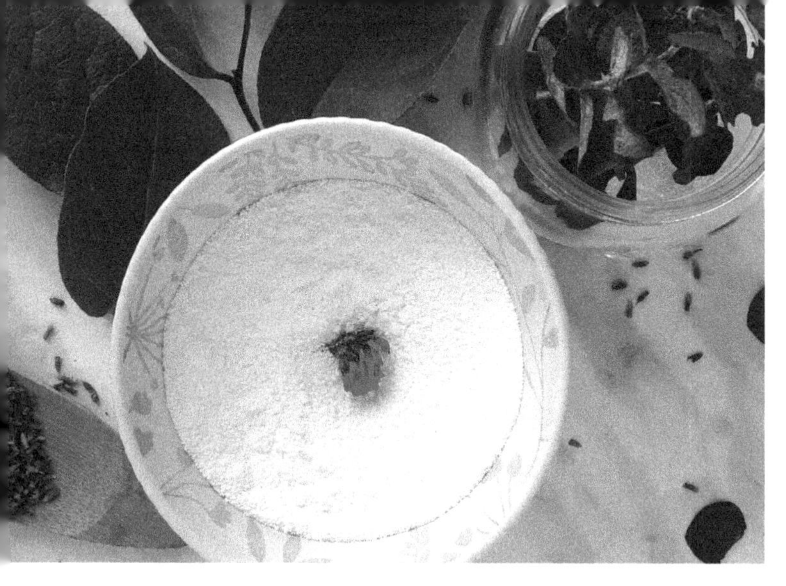

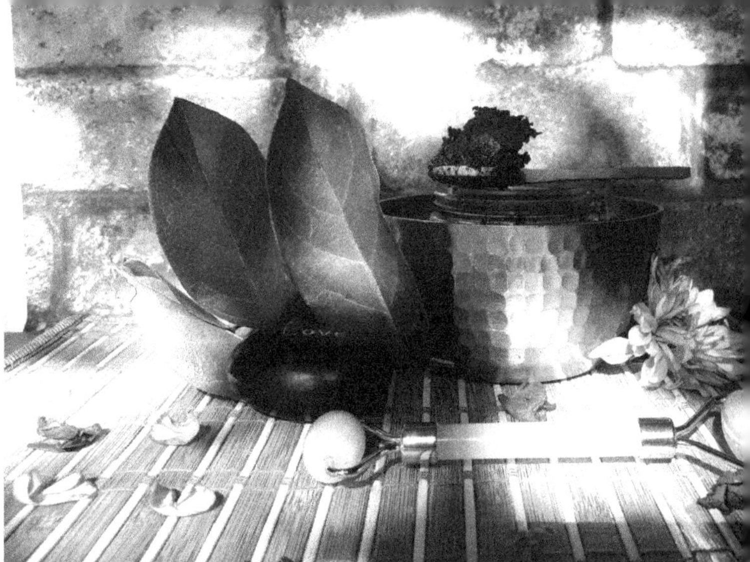

Dedicated to you, mom

Apothecary – an ancient term meaning drugstore or pharmacy. It is also the investigation of herbal and chemical ingredients, and preparation of a product.

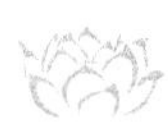

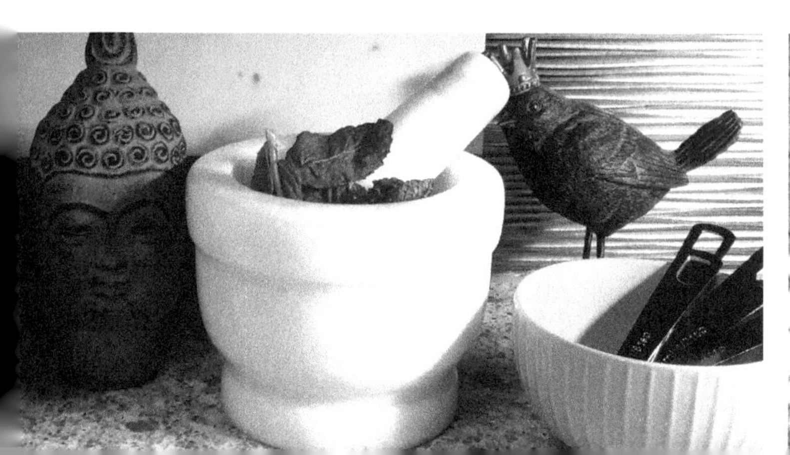

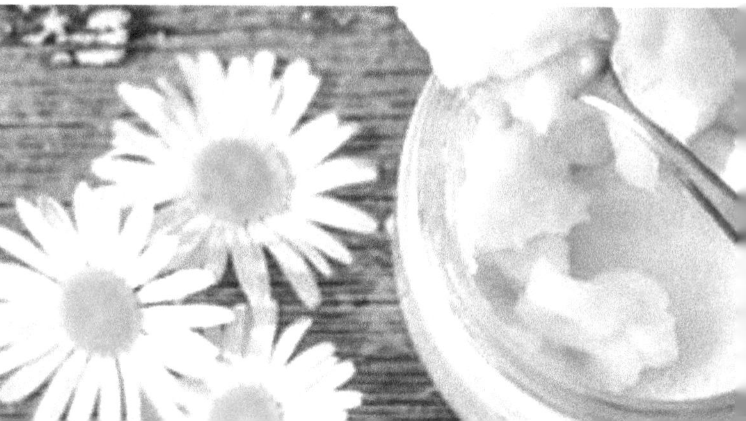

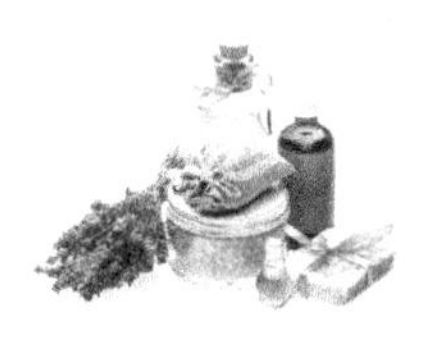

Table of Contents

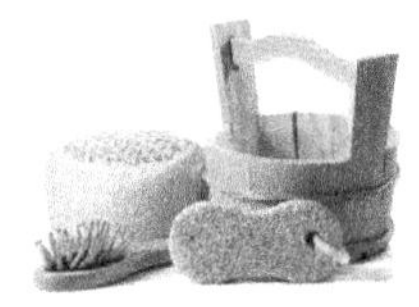

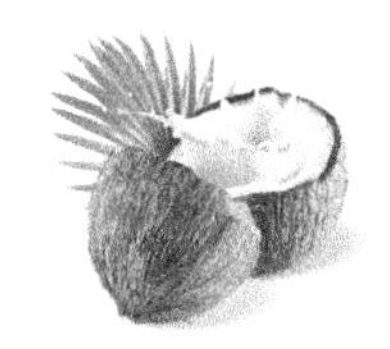
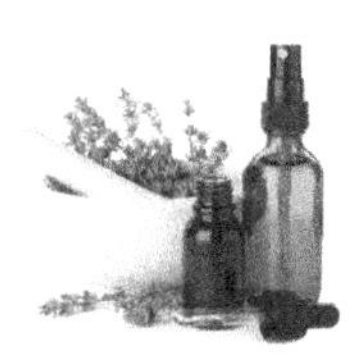
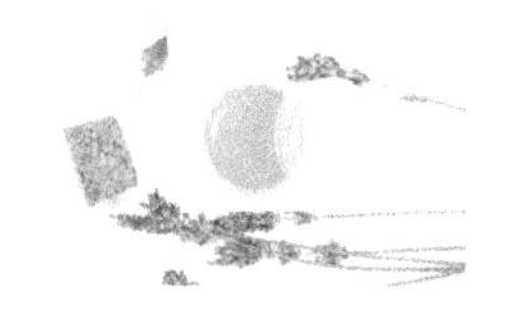
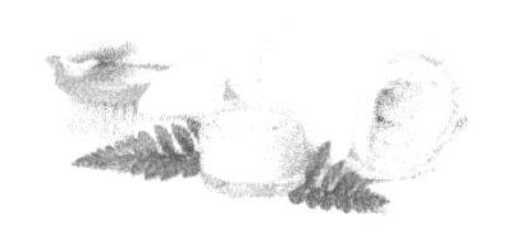

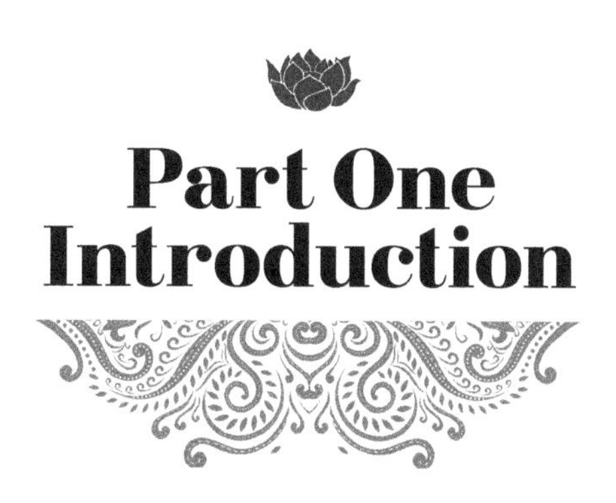

Part One
Introduction

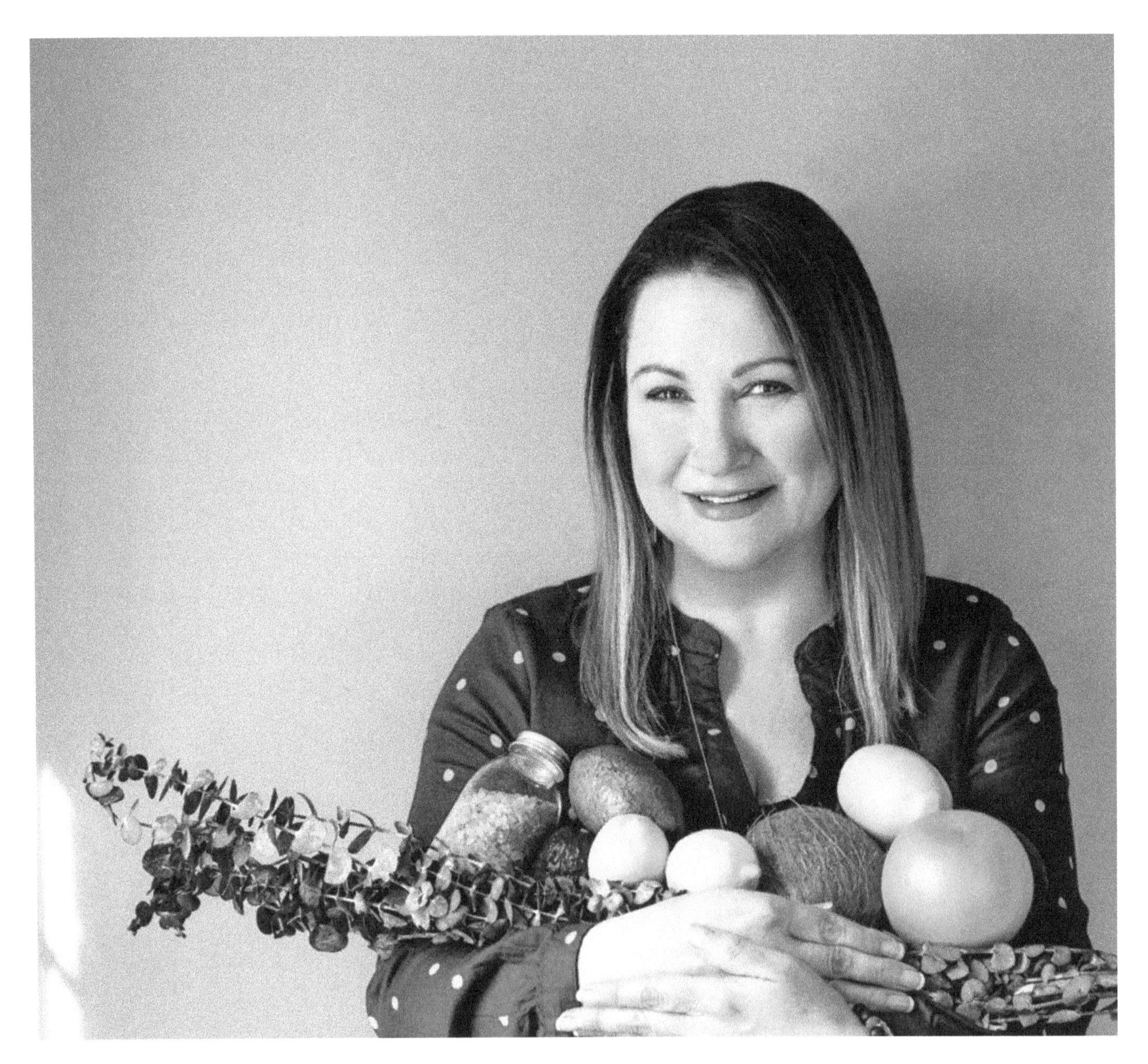

PHOTO CREDIT: **NAT CARON**

MY STORY

As a child I always had a sensitive immune system. A low-birth-weight baby with a history of respiratory infections and chronic colds, I missed a lot of school because of my ailments. But all the pediatrician could do was *give* me antibiotics. I was on antibiotics at least twice a year. As we now understand, over-prescribing can cause antibiotic resistance. In my twenties I began searching for alternative ways to cure myself. Thus began my fascination and curiosity with holistic medicine.

A big shift in my world came when I had my first child in 1999. Becoming a mother changes everything, especially your perspective. I now had this new life to care for and I took my responsibility seriously. This is where my obsession with reading labels came into play. It sure takes a lot longer to get the shopping done, but I certainly didn't want to give my baby anything *unnatural*. My son unfortunately inherited my asthma and susceptibility to viruses – and a severe allergy to all nuts. Therefore, even more careful investigation of safe foods and products was necessary.

In an era of plastics, pollution, pesticides, and genetically modified food (known as GMOs or genetically modified organisms), it's often difficult to navigate what is safe to consume. That is why I began making everything from scratch for my kids, as I still do today.

The best way to know what's in your food is to make it yourself.

Aromatherapy is another area I wanted to explore further. I had been interested in essential oils back in the 1990s, and this time I took it to a new level – I became a certified aromatherapist. It's such a gift to be able to use these healing oils for a variety of causes. Our medicine cabinet now brims with lavender oil and tea tree oil, instead of over-the-counter medications.

In late 2017, I began to experiment with making my own natural products from home. I started out with just a few balms here and there. Suddenly, my sister wanted me to make her a body powder and a friend needed a pain-relieving salve. That's how my company, Lark & the Lotus, was born. We now make a full range of body butters, tinctures, balms, and bath products – our very own healing apothecary – and I'm excited to share this knowledge with you!

Helping people shift from commercial products to all-natural ones has been the most gratifying experience. Giving them knowledge to also create their own *green and clean* home feels like the next step. And so, the idea of a DIY (do-it-yourself) book arose organically, through educating and demonstrating how DIY is easy and affordable – and not to mention FUN! My recipes have been tried, tested, and reformulated again, and sometimes again. I hope you enjoy this book as much as I enjoyed writing it.

As I often say, **it's easier than whipping up a batch of cookies!** This is my gift to you and, in turn, your gift to your own family. I truly believe the earth is equipped with plants that can heal our bodies and minds, so we can live the healthiest life possible.

It feels great, and you are worth the effort!

Susan

PHOTO CREDIT: **NAT CARON**

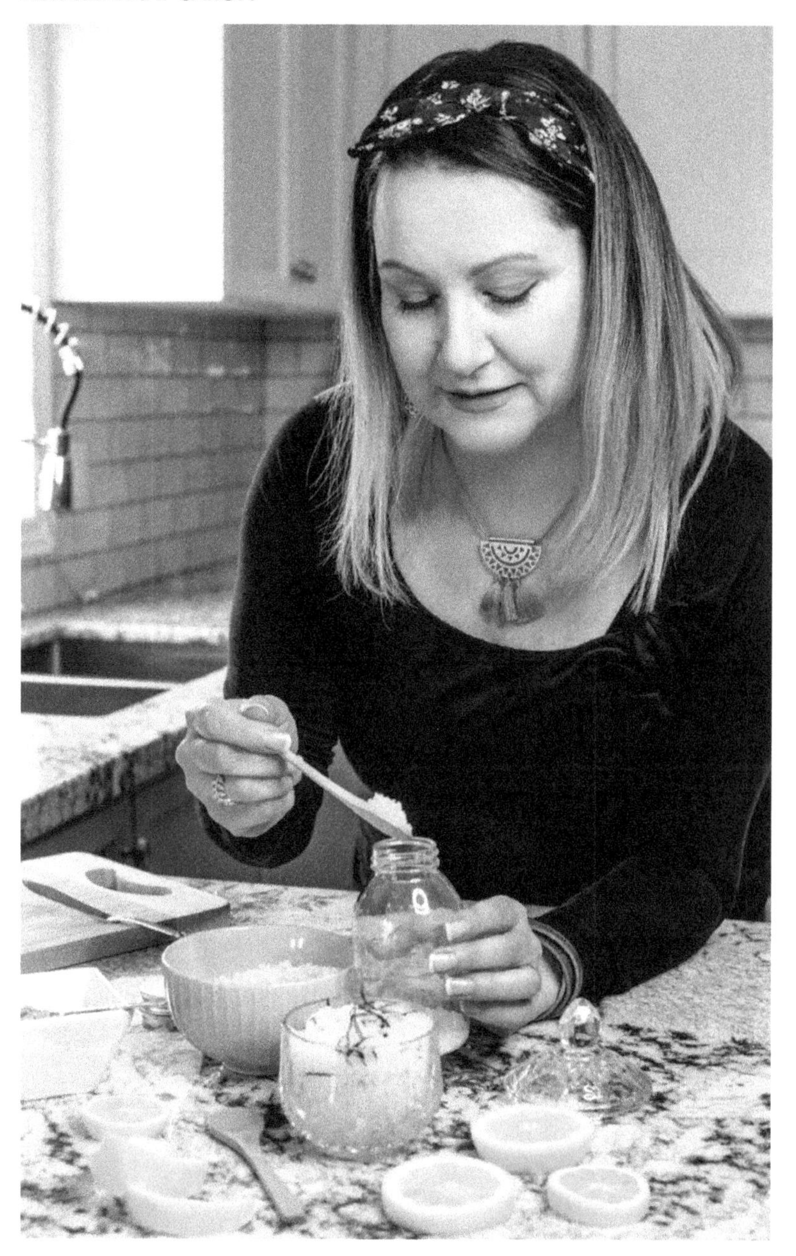

WHY DIY?
Understanding the Benefits

You may be thinking: I don't have time to DIY; it's easier to just buy off the shelf. You are right. It *is* easier to buy off the shelf, but it isn't *better* or safer to do so. How I became a DIYer is simple. I didn't like what I was seeing on the store shelves. Although the packaging looked pretty and it smelled lovely, I'm the type of person who *reads the label.* If you read the label on your products, you'll be astounded at what you find. Even in the so-called "natural" products, you may come across ingredients that don't sound very natural. Basically, I had a hard time trusting what was in the products and what I would be putting on the largest organ in my body – my skin. I also had my children to think of. What about their health? This prompted me to do a lot of research to find out what I was really using each day.

There is a fine line between what is toxic and what is deemed safe for use. In the cosmetic industry, small amounts of chemicals are allowed to be added to our merchandise. Although, these might be minute additions, who is taking into consideration how often we should apply these? For most of us, we like a routine. This means we normally use the same shampoo and conditioner each day, mop the floor with the same solution, and so on. These chemicals build up over time, causing a toxic overload in our homes, environment, and ultimately our bodies.

Chemicals are added to our products for a number of reasons.

Preservatives: to preserve the product and give it a longer shelf life
Thickeners: to thicken the product
Surfactants: to make the product foam
Synthetic fragrance: to enhance the smell
Emulsifiers: to prevent ingredients from separating
Artificial colourants: to add colour

In order to take control of what I was applying to my body, I decided to create my own bath and body essentials. I am pleased to say I have greatly reduced the commercial chemicals in my home for over a decade. I no longer need to buy box-store toothpaste, deodorant, body cream, or bath products because I make my own. Not only do I save a lot of money, I have peace of mind knowing exactly what goes into each container. I choose organic, vegan, high-quality ingredients, and 100% therapeutic-grade organic essential oils.

For this book, I have covered mainly bath and body products – from lip balms to moisturizers, body spray, and bath wash; products for babies and kids; and fun spa-day masks and scrubs. I will save the home cleaning and cosmetic DIYs for a subsequent edition, so stay tuned!

If you are looking to improve your health, save money, and create a chemical-free environment, you've come to the right place.

This book contains easy, step-by-step instructions on how to DIY your own personal-care items. Every recipe is plant-based, cruelty-free, as organic as possible, and always chemical-free. The recipes can be customized to add scent or keep unscented.

I've also included ideas for containing and embellishing your lovely creations. You'll be DIYing like a pro in no time!

WHAT'S IN YOUR PRODUCTS?

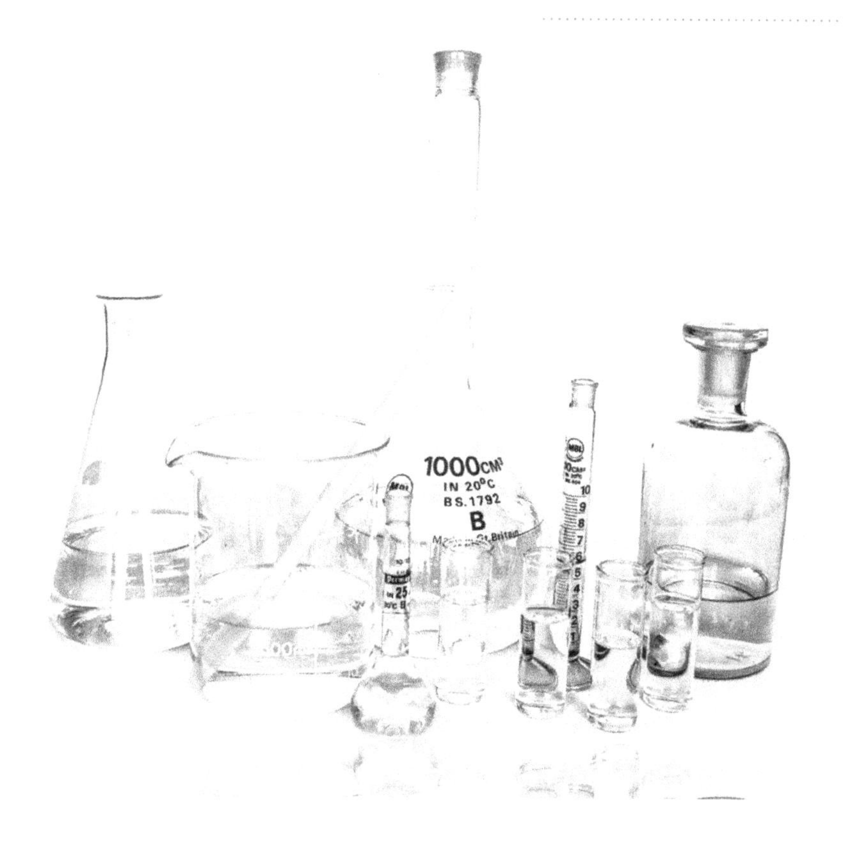

Would you spray anti-freeze on your body? Or rub coal on your baby's delicate skin?

We all answered, "No way!" But unfortunately, we *are* already putting these types of chemicals on our bodies every day. Baby products are no exception in the manufacturing world.

Did you know, on average, women apply approximately ten products on their bodies each day? Imagine how many chemicals this adds up to.

I encourage you to have a look at the ingredients listed on your cosmetics, cleaners, and bath-and-body product labels. What you'll see is a lot of scientific names that sound very sci-fi and unnatural.

As we are learning, cosmetics are filled with *many* harmful chemicals. As consumers, we are covering our bodies from head to toe each day with toxins.

Health-compromising ingredients you will commonly see listed in your products are aluminum, dioxane, dyes, formaldehyde, fragrance, parabens, petroleum, phthalates, sodium lauryl sulfate, and talc. Even the so-called natural products will list "fragrance," and some type of preservative.

Aerosols are particularly hazardous to the environment and ozone layer. An aerosol takes a liquid, such as hairspray, and turns it into a fine mist. To do this, it requires a propellant chemical called "butane." Other products that use a propellant include shaving creams, sprayable sunscreen, and body and room sprays. These are products you *definitely* want to avoid using.

Fragrance is a chemical cocktail that causes a variety of health problems but is allowed to be sold to consumers. There is a trade-secret agreement that allows manufacturers to withhold the ingredient list from the public. They can add *literally anything* they want to the so-called trade-secret fragrance, and that is what's most alarming. Fragrances can cause a range of side-effects from headaches to nausea, dizziness, itching, and allergies.

Sounds crazy, I know! You may ask, "How and why are these items allowed to be sold to us?" Good question, but sadly in North America they *are* allowed.

Every country has a different set of laws. In Europe for instance, they have banned approximately 1,300 chemicals from personal products. Canada has banned about 600 chemicals, and the United States has only banned about 30 chemicals. Those are frightening statistics.

So, what can we do?

For now, we must advocate for ourselves and decide what we want to purchase. Education is key. The more we know, the better we can promote health for ourselves and our families Remember, just because it's being sold in a store doesn't make it safe to use. I've compiled data from the Environmental Working Group (EWG) and, more specifically, from their Skin Deep database. EWG is an American non-profit, non-partisan organization dedicated to protecting our health and environment. On their website, you can search a brand name or any ingredient you read on your label and find out more. The chemicals are listed from low to high toxicity. You can check out the database at ewg.org/skindeep.

In Canada there is a Cosmetic Ingredient Hotlist that outlines which chemicals are prohibited and which are restricted. Go to canada.ca/en/health-canada/services/cosmetics.html.

I've listed the most hazardous chemicals found in our bath and body products. No doubt you've heard of some of these, but now you'll learn just what they're about.

Ingredient	Other names	Where found	Side effects
Acrylamide		Cosmetics	Linked to cancer
Artificial fragrance	Parfum, linalool, phthalates	Cosmetics, body cream, bath products	Allergic reactions, headaches, dizziness, skin irritation
Butane		Hair spray, shaving foam, body spray, sunscreen spray	Eye and skin irritant Can affect organs Harmful to environment
Butylated hydroxytoluene	BHT	Perfume, body spray, fragrance	Allergies, cancer, endocrine disruption, immunotoxicity, irritation, reproductive and organ system toxicity
Cetylpyridinium chloride		Used as an antistatic, antimacrobial	Allergic reactions, immunotoxicity
Distearyldimonium chloride		Hair products	Skin irritation
DMDM hydantoin		In about 20% of personal care products and cosmetics	Allergies, cancer, reproductive problems, skin irritation Releases formaldehyde

1,4-Dioxane	Myreth, oleth, laureth, ceteareth	In almost 50% of cosmetics Made with petroleum-derived ethylene oxide	One of the most harmful chemicals Known carcinogen linked to cancers, birth defects
Formaldehyde		Nail polish, nail products	Known carcinogen
Methylchloroisothiazolinone	2-methyl-3(2H)-isothiazolone,	Preservative in hair/bath/body products, cosmetics	Cancer, skin and eye irritation
Mineral oil	Petrolatum, liquid petroleum, liquid paraffin	Petroleum-derived substance in cosmetics, baby products, body lotion	Linked to increased estrogen production
Oxybenzone	Phenyl-methanone, 2-hydroxy-4-methoxyphenyl	UV light absorber/filter in sunscreen	Endocrine disruption, organ toxicity
Paraben	Methyl, propyl, butyl, ethyl	Preservative in cosmetics, skin cream, deodorant	Found in breast tissue Linked to breast cancer
Palm oil	Palm kernel oil, palmitate, sodium laureth, sodium lauryl, sorbitan, steareth, stearic acid, stearyl, TEA	In most hair products, body products, cosmetics	Linked to tumour growth, cancer Harvesting linked to deforestation, destruction of orangutans
Petrolatum	Paraffin, dipropylene, glycol, butylene glycol, disodium EDTA, tetrasodium EDTA, polybutene, triclosan, polyethylene	Petroleum-derived substance used as a skin barrier to keep skin moist and conditioned	Linked to tumour growth Linked to increased estrogen production Blocks pores, preventing the skin from breathing Can cause acne and breakouts

Phthalates	dibutyl phthalate, diethylhexyl phthalate	Fragrance and plasticizer in skin care products, shampoo, makeup, deodorant, nail polish	Can damage kidneys, liver, lungs, reproductive system
Propylene Glycol	Polyethylene Glycol (PEG)	Derived from the same chemical that makes anti-freeze	Easily penetrates skin Can damage kidney, liver, brain
Silicone	Cyclomethicone, dimethicone, copolyol, phenyl trimethicone	Smoothing and thickening agent in shampoo, skin cream	Linked to tumours
Styrene	Benzene, ethenyl, ethenylbenzene	Fragrance in baby soap, body wash, sunscreen	Endocrine disruption, cancer, developmental/ reproductive toxicity
Synthetic colour	FD&C, D&C	Colourant in cosmetics, nail polish, hair dye, bath products Some colourants derived from coal tar, containing toxic heavy metals	
Talc	Talcum	Moisture-absorbing agent in baby powder, blush, makeup	Linked to ovarian cancer Can contain asbestos
Triclosan	5-chloro-2, phenol	Cosmetic biocide, preservative and antibacterial agent in personal care and cleaning products	May be associated with endocrine (hormonal) toxicity

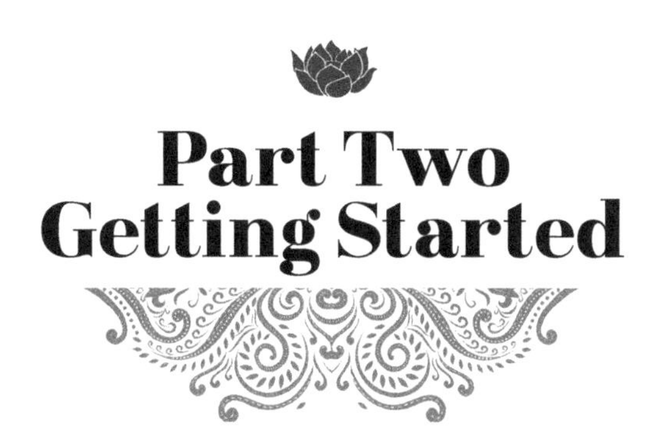

Part Two
Getting Started

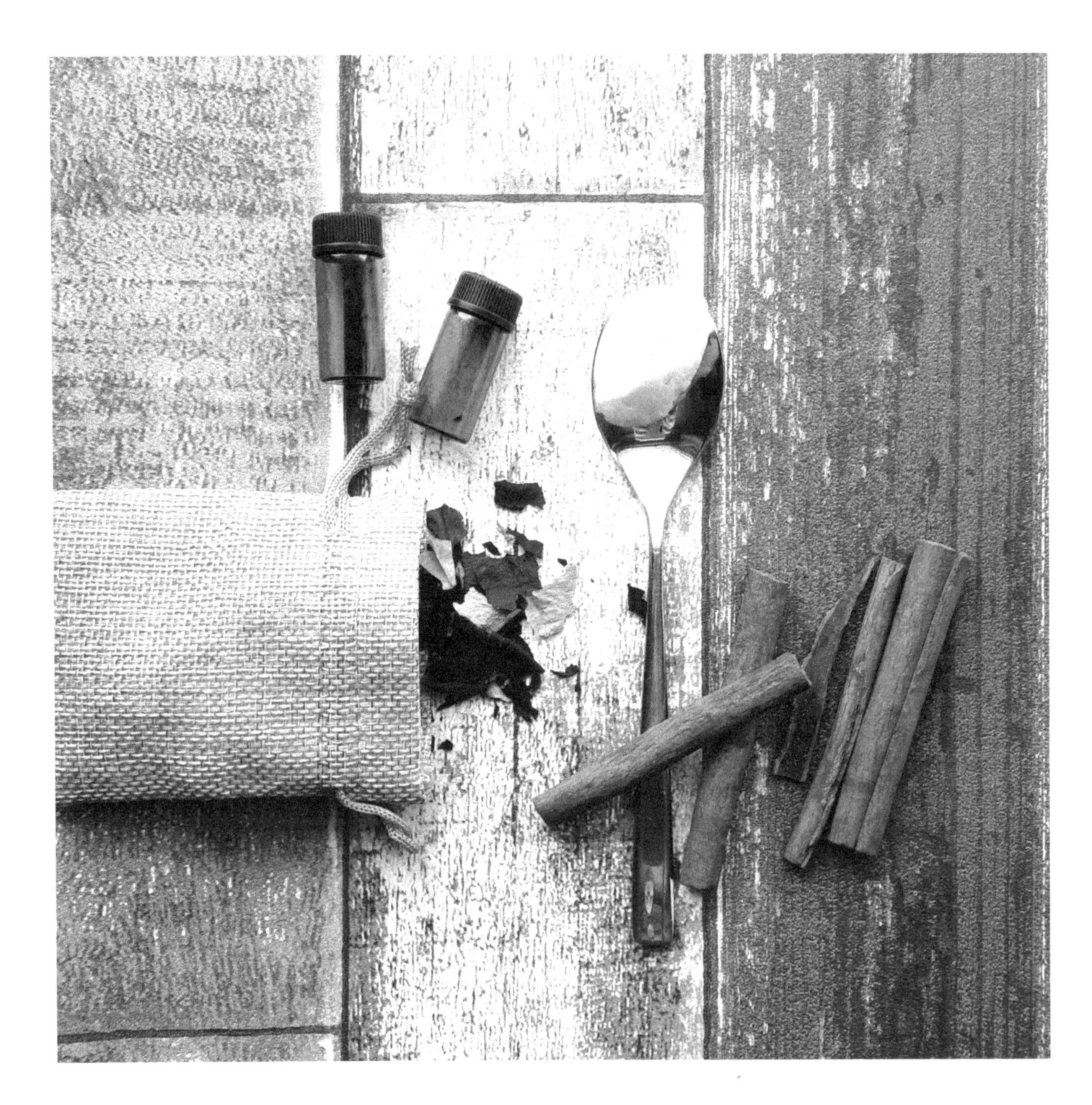

ALL-NATURAL INGREDIENTS
My Natural Toolkit

My all-natural tool-kit consists of a few key ingredients that you can literally eat; that's how natural they are! You can find these in your local health food store or grocery store's health aisle.

Organic coconut oil – a semi-hard oil and staple for skin and body care. Coconut oil has many uses. It is antibacterial, anti-inflammatory, and helpful for acne. It can be a bit pricey, so do shop around.

Liquid coconut oil – a liquid version of organic coconut oil with many versatile uses. This oil will not harden and is used in many lotions.

Avocado oil – a deeply nourishing oil rich in fatty acids and containing vitamin E. Perfect for body butters and moisturizers.

Organic shea butter – high in fatty acids and an anti-inflammatory. For best results, shop for the unscented version.

Cocoa butter – a wonderful-smelling, rich, moisturizing butter. I prefer the raw, unrefined version for the full aroma, but it is also available refined (unscented).

Beeswax – can be found at local craft stores in a brick shape or as pellets, which are easier for melting. Beeswax gives products firmness and is especially good for lip balms. If you use brick beeswax, you will need to grate it with a cheese grater first.

Pure extracts – can add natural flavours to lip products. When choosing extracts always look for pure, organic, and clear liquid. Note that vanilla extract does not blend nicely in products; therefore, I recommend using vanilla stevia for that vanilla flavour.

Grapeseed oil – an inexpensive all-purpose carrier oil. It is light in colour and odourless, and will not tint your lotions.

Jojoba oil – another great carrier oil. It contains vitamins B and E, and is very moisturizing. It also has a rich golden colour. I prefer this oil in skin creams and bath products.

Liquid castile soap – contains the least amount of chemicals. I recommend an unscented version so you can add your own essential oils. Castile soap is suitable for hand soap and shower gels.

Organic beet root powder – provides a gorgeous purple-red colour that can be used to naturally tint your lip balms, glosses, bath bombs, etc. It also has anti-aging and antioxidant benefits.

Organic cocoa powder – adds a lovely scent and colour to lip balms and body products. It contains many antioxidants too.

Matcha green tea powder – a natural earthy colourant full of healing antioxidants. It has a mild, pleasant aroma.

Liquid stevia – a plant-based, sugar-free, chemical-free sweetener that's perfect for lip balms when you want to add some flavour. You can also find flavoured stevia, such as chocolate, vanilla, and hazelnut. They make for great-tasting lip products.

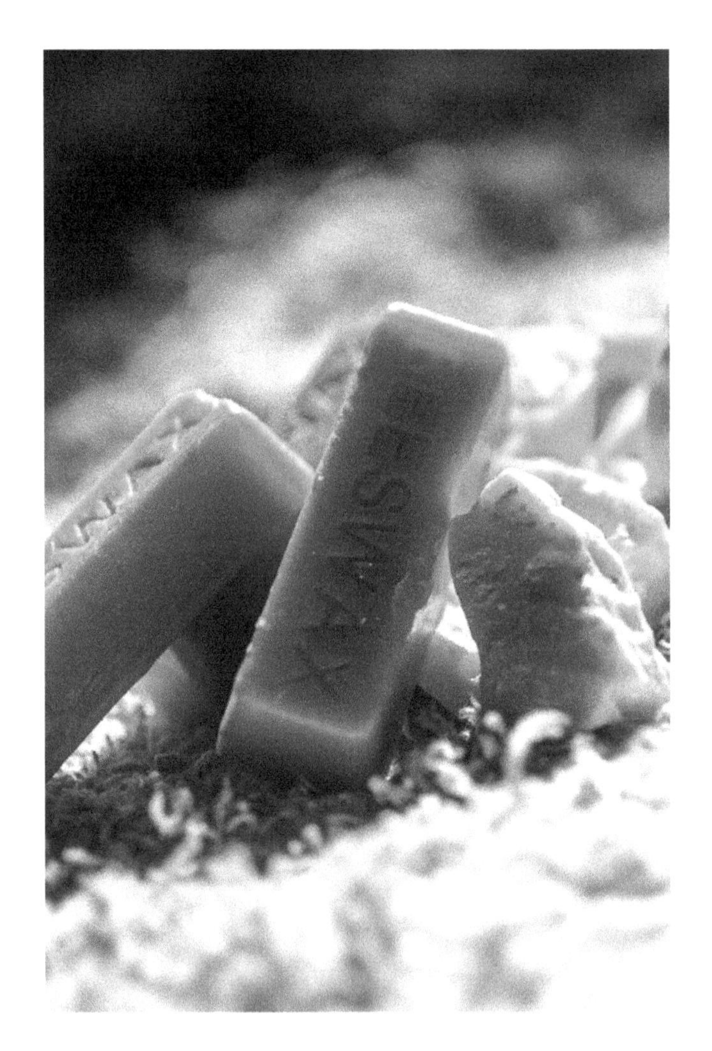

Honey – adds natural flavour to lip products and is also an antioxidant. I prefer to use local honey to support our beekeepers.

Vitamin E oil – great for the skin, wound healing, and scar reduction. It also serves as a natural preservative, helping products last longer. I like to add vitamin E oil to lip balm and body products. Don't skip on vitamin E.

Essential oils – add natural scent to your products and have many healing benefits. By using only 100% therapeutic-grade essential oils, you'll receive only the good stuff. So why don't manufacturers just use essential oils, you may wonder? Because the scent of these oils is not as strong as commercial fragrances and doesn't last as long. Not to mention, the oils are more expensive than synthetic fragrance. Making your own fresh products will help ensure months of enjoyment.

Please note, I do not endorse any particular product or company, so I recommend you shop around for the best prices for ingredients. Coconut and avocado oils tend to be pricey. You can find most ingredients in your local health food store and supermarket. You can also check online stores such as **Amazon**. There are some great price-comparing apps to check out like **Flipp** and **Flyerify**.

The ingredients I use are all plant-based and cruelty-free, and some recipes contain honey and beeswax. If you have an issue with using any of the ingredients, you will need to find a substitute. Honey can be omitted or replaced with agave or stevia sweetener. Beeswax, however, is a key component to solidify the product and must be replaced with candelilla wax. Please note, candelilla is denser, so the recipe will need to be modified to accommodate this.

Keep in mind, if you are changing the recipe, the results will vary.

Many people ask if it's alright to use mica powder as a colourant. Mica is derived from a group of naturally occurring minerals and appears shimmery. I don't recommend *coloured* mica powder because it contains pigment. If you see the word "pigment" on the label, it is not natural.

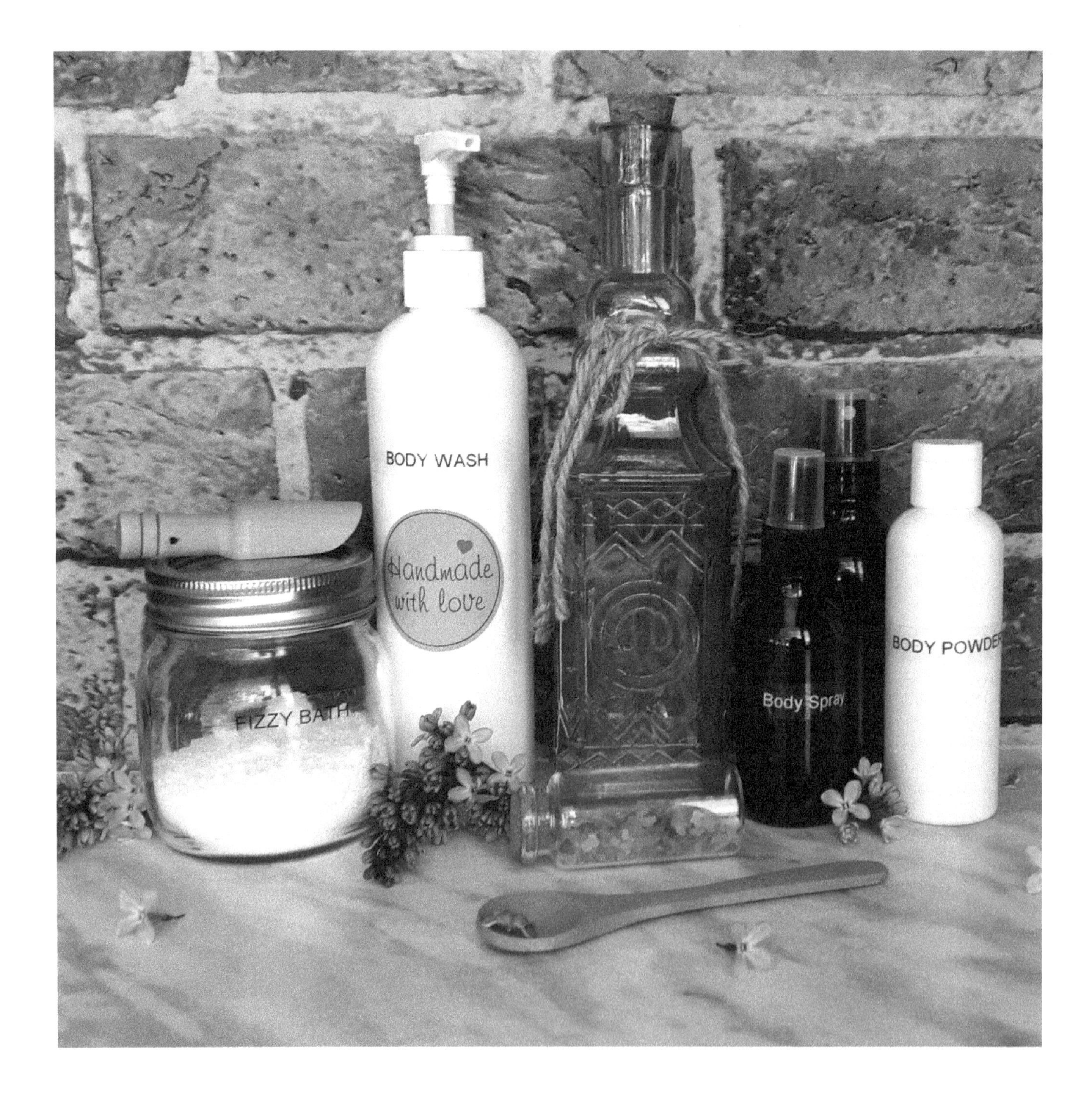
BODY WASH
Handmade with love
FIZZY BATH
Body Spray

PACKAGING
How to Show Off Your Creations

Packaging containers hold and display your lovely creations. When sourcing a suitable container, we recommend glass or recyclable plastic. Glass is a good choice because it's easy to clean, recyclable, and better for the environment. Plastic is not environmentally friendly, as it does not decompose with time and fills up our landfills, lakes, and oceans. If you use plastic containers, check to see if they are recyclable. The two types of containers you'll come across are PET (polyethylene terephthalate) and HDPE (high-density polyethylene). These are made from recycled materials and can be recycled again. Look for containers that are BPA (bisphenol A) free. BPA is a xenoestrogen, which is known to disrupt hormones in humans.

Pictured here are the types of containers you can use for your products. You don't have to spend a lot for practical storage. You'll find a wide variety, from small sample-size containers, which are great for lip glosses and travelling, to larger glass containers for balms and scrubs, in the craft section of the Dollar Store, Walmart, and Michaels. Again, look for the *recycle symbol* and the words "BPA free."

Mason jars are another great item to have on hand. They come in a variety of shapes and sizes, and you can use them again and again. You can find unique containers for lip balms and glosses on Amazon. The bamboo containers are a bit pricey but look amazing! They make a great gift too.

Reusing your old containers is a good idea. Less waste is always good news for the planet. Just be sure to clean and sanitize them first to kill any bacteria.

Find fun ways to store and share your creations.

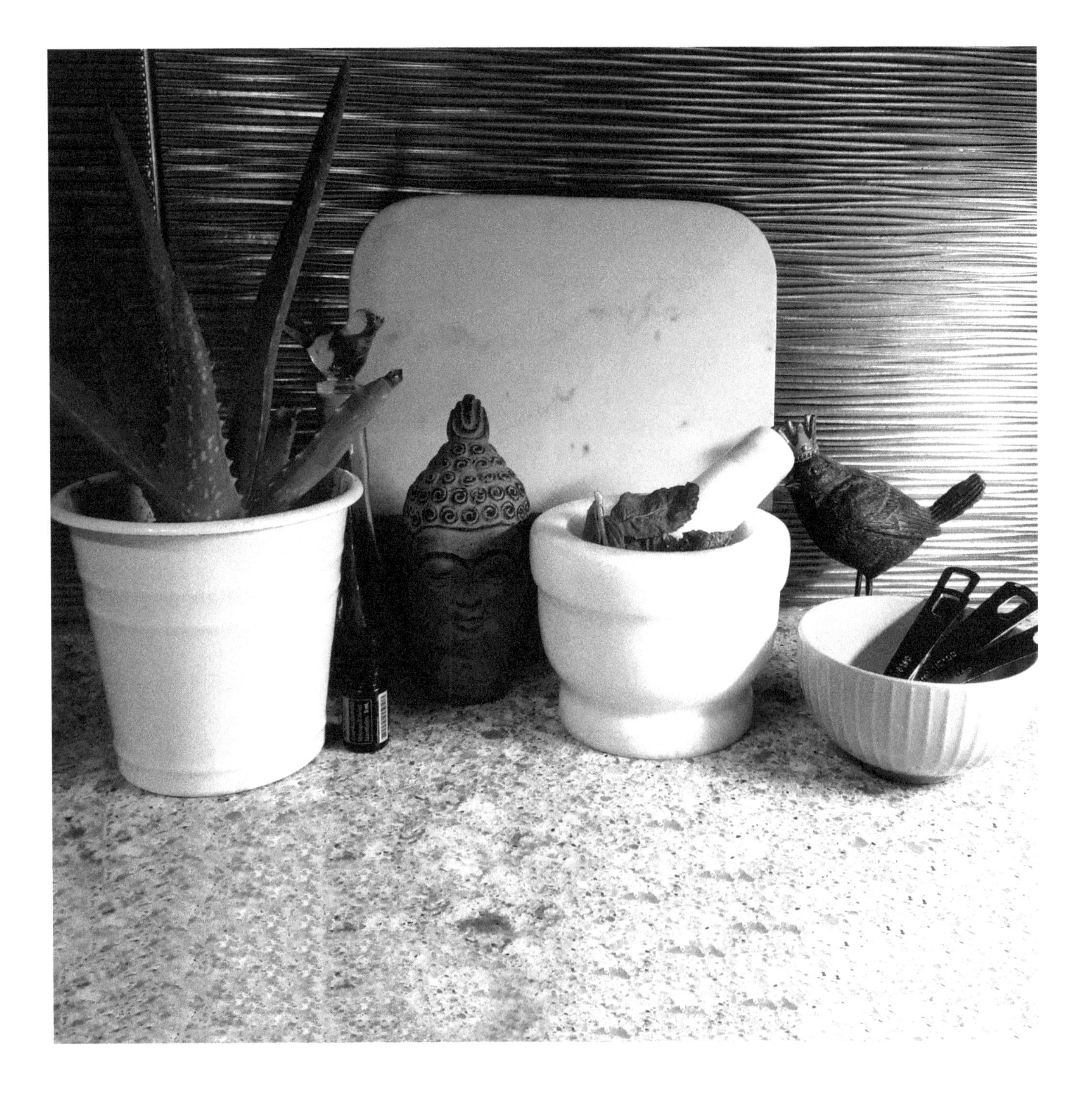

EQUIPMENT

What You'll Need to Prepare Before You Start

Are you ready to take the plunge and make your own products? Before you begin, there are a few things you'll need to prepare.

The kitchen is the best place to make your items. Be sure to wash your counters down because you don't want crumbs in your balms, right? Wipe down your stovetop, microwave, and so on.

There are two heating methods you can use – microwave or stove top. The recipes will show specific instructions for each heating type.

I suggest using a large, clean cutting board as your work area. You will also need the following items:

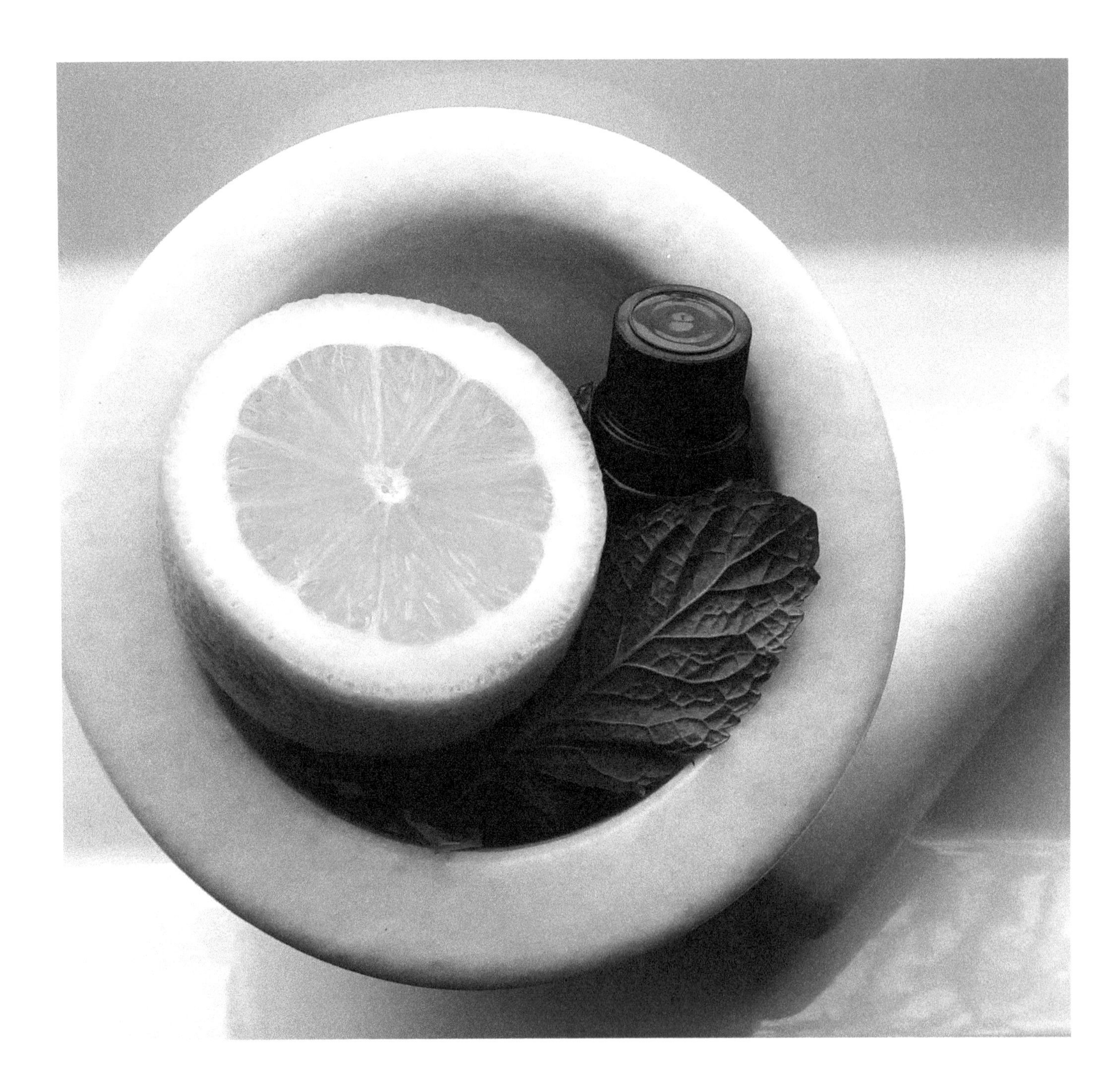

- 2 cup Pyrex glass measuring cups or a large mason jar
- Set of measuring cups
- Set of measuring spoons
- Fine metal strainer or tea strainer
- Food processor
- Mortar and pestle or mini chopper
- Metal spoon for stirring
- Zester or grater
- Clean tea towels
- Clean, dry containers for each recipe

You may also wish to use a pair of heat-resistant gloves. I say gloves and not oven mitts because you need to properly grip the measuring cup to pour. Oven mitts are too bulky, which can result in more accidents.

Safe for kids? I don't recommend these recipes for kids under 12 unless supervised by an adult. When dealing with scalding hot liquid, why take a chance? It's certainly fun for kids to participate, so find other jobs for them to do while keeping them involved but safe.

Have your containers ready for use as well. Be sure they are clean, dry, and ready to be poured into. I suggest removing the lids and placing them in another location. Place the containers on the clean cutting board to catch drips and spills. If you drip any product onto the cutting board, allow it to cool slightly and reuse.

Next: Select the recipe you wish to use and then set out the ingredients, essential oils, and containers you will need.

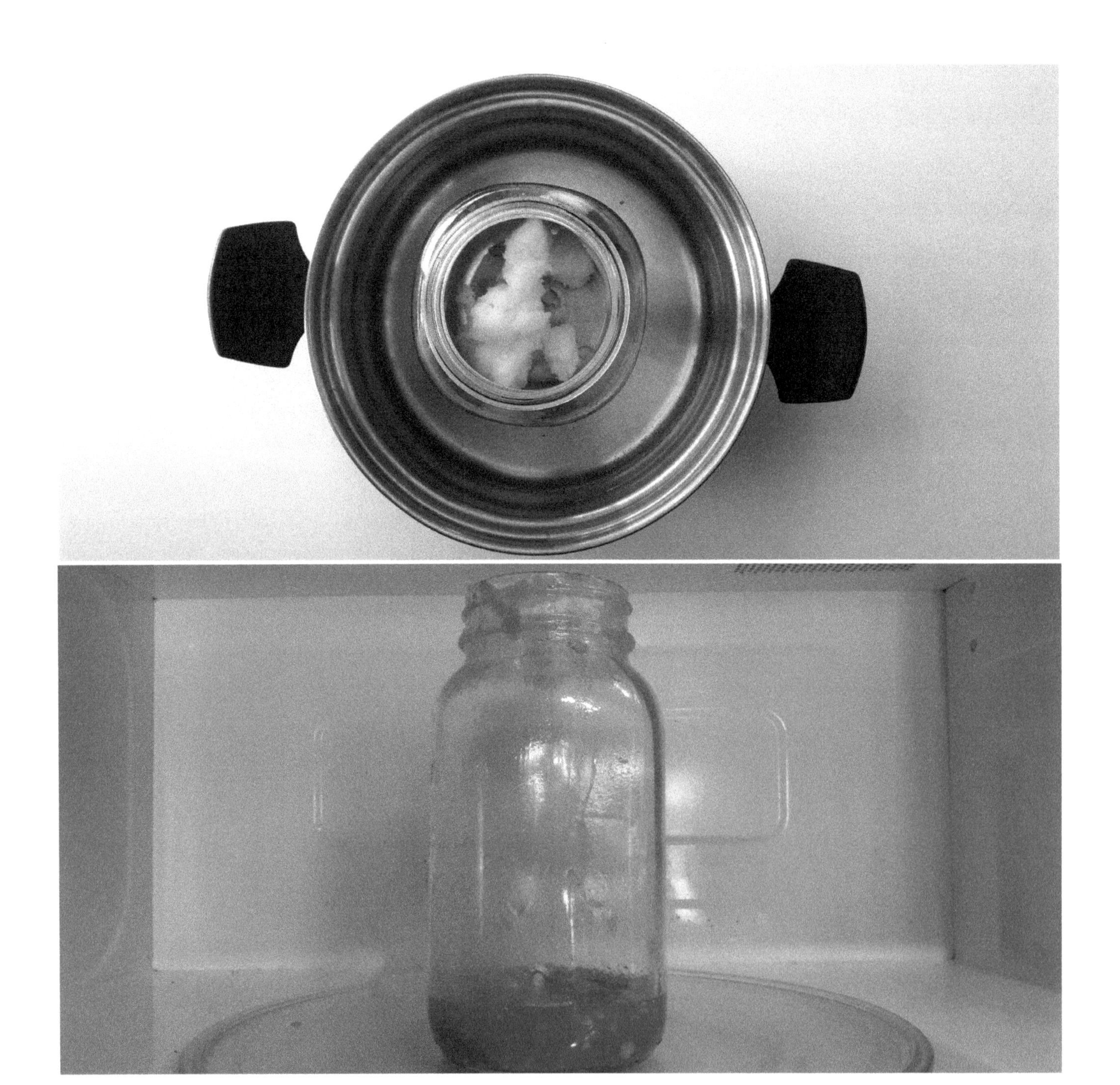

HEATING AND POURING

All of these recipes require the melting of oil, butters, and/or wax (raw materials) together. This process is safe and easy, and you can choose whichever method you prefer. The end results are exactly the same.

The quickest and cleanest method is with a microwave. It will take under five minutes to melt your raw materials.

If you are using a microwave, you will need a glass measuring cup or mason jar. You will be heating in 30-second intervals to avoid overheating and scorching ingredients.

Do not heat essential oils in the microwave. Add these last, once your other ingredients are melted. Cooking the essential oils can damage their integrity.

For the stovetop method, you will create a double boiler with a pot and a glass measuring cup. This method uses a low-medium heat to gently melt the oils.

Add 2 to 3 cold cups of water to the pot. The water should reach halfway up the glass cup or jar. Do not get water *in* the jar.

It takes about 15 minutes to completely melt the raw materials.

Always use caution when removing the glass cup from the pot of hot water.

Remember to add essential oils last and do not heat them.

Tips: If you accidentally pour melted oils onto your skin, wipe them off immediately with a towel and run your hand under cool water. Try some aloe vera gel, as it cools skin quickly. A heat-safe glove is recommended when handling hot liquid.

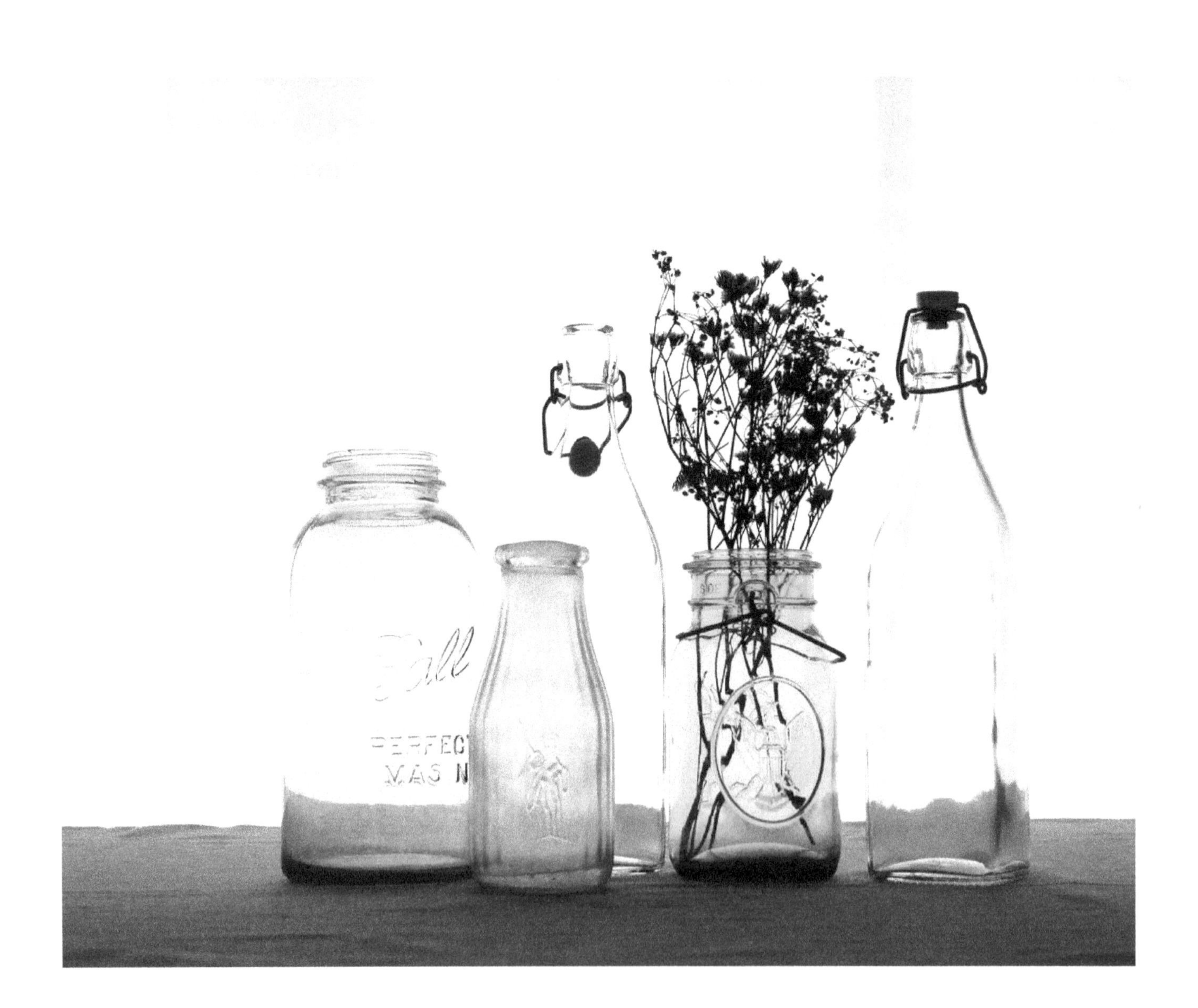

EASY CLEAN-UP

Most of the recipes involve oils, butters, and/or waxes that harden when cooled. For easy clean-up, here are a few suggestions.

- Scrape any hardened butters and waxes into a container to reuse again or discard in your food-waste compost bin.
- Avoid pouring melted product down your kitchen sink drain. You risk an eventual clog within your pipes.
- When using a dishwasher, ensure your pots and glass jars do not have any remaining wax or butter product because this will melt and eventually clog up your dishwasher pipes.
- If you get oils onto your clothing, you should treat this right away, before it sets into a permanent stain. First, try to soak up as much oil as possible with a towel or paper towel. Then pour baking soda onto the area and leave for 10 to 15 minutes. Lastly, try a little dish soap to wash out the remaining oil.

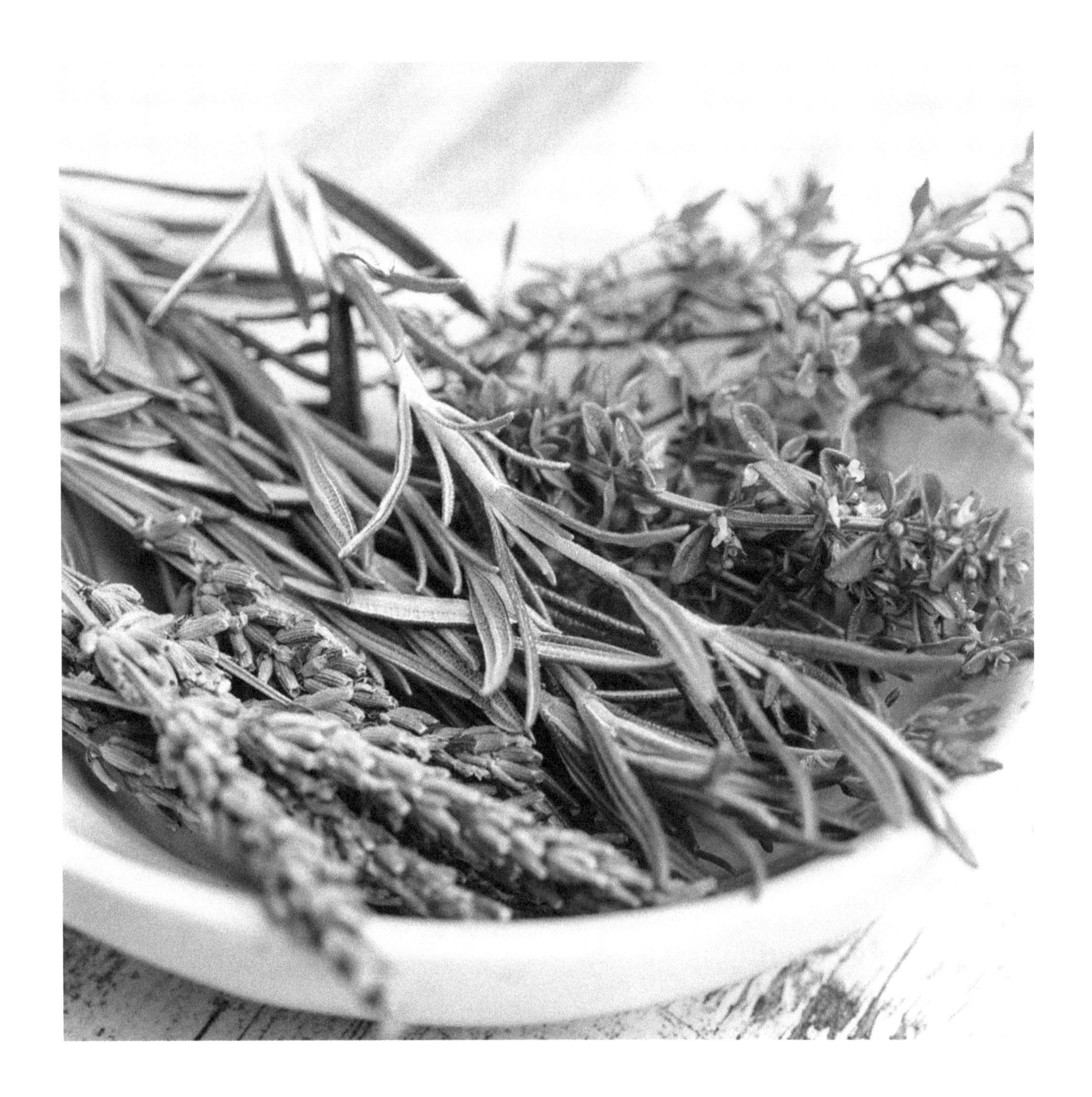

ABOUT THE RECIPES

I've made the recipes as simple as possible. There are no fancy ingredients and no complicated instructions. You don't need to be a cook to follow these tutorials. Simply scooping raw materials into measuring cups and spoons, and warming ingredients is all that's required. We're not all chefs, I know! Quick and simple is the objective here.

Be sure to read the **Tips** on the recipe page before you begin to ensure a successful end- product.

The recipes can be modified to suit you. For instance, if you want to make more or less of the product, you can half or double the recipe. If you prefer a firmer product, add a tablespoon more beeswax. If you prefer a softer, creamier result, add a tablespoon more coconut oil.

The scents are customizable to your personal preferences. I have suggested a moderate amount of essential oil, but I suggest you smell the mixture and add more essential oils as needed. The rule of thumb is 2% of essential oils can be added to any product. Keep in mind that once the essential oils are mixed in the product, it has about a one-month shelf life and the scent will begin to fade within that timeframe. So, a mixture that smells strong today, will eventually lessen.

Flavours have been suggested for a minimal sweetness – nothing overpowering or sickly-sweet here. You can taste the mixture while it's melted and add more stevia and extracts as you see fit. The bottom line is, **it has to be right for you**.

Tip: If you keep your completed project in the fridge, the shelf life will increase to about three months.

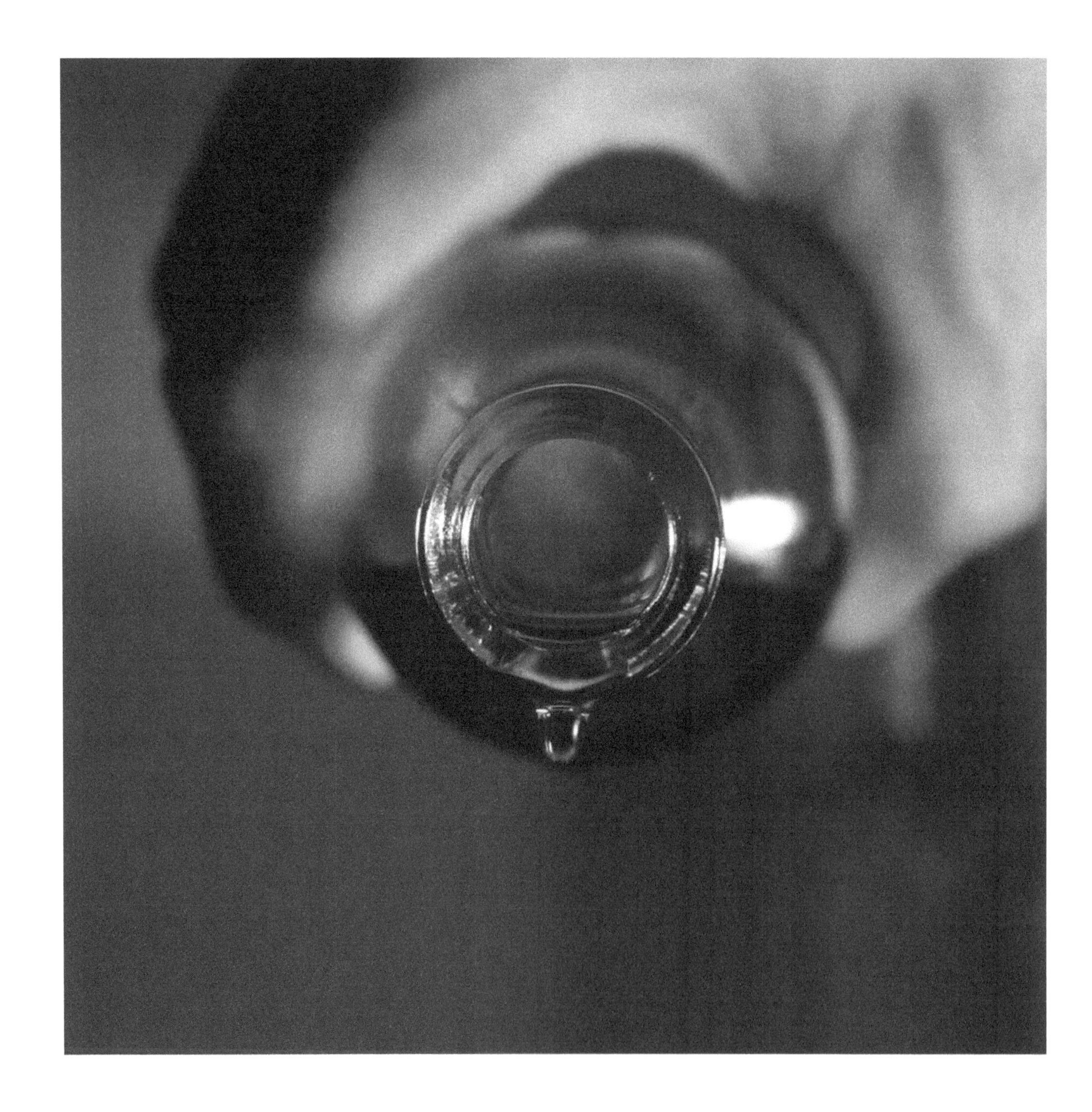

ESSENTIAL OIL KNOW-HOW
Everything You Need to Know

You may have noticed that essential oils are quite trendy these days, with cool mist diffusers, diffuser jewelry, and more! Essential oils are not new; in fact, they've been around a long, long time. Ancient Egyptians used essential oils as perfume, medicine and embalming methods. We now call the practice aromatherapy, as there are many healing therapies from its use. Essential oils are derived from plants, seeds, peels, and wood. Distillation is the purest way of obtaining the precious oils.

The essential oils we recommend are 100% pure and don't have to be expensive. Just ensure they are pure and for therapeutic use. Essential oils can be volatile on their own, so never apply them directly onto the skin without diluting. You can dilute the oils two ways: add them to water for diffusing in the air or to a carrier oil to be applied to the skin.

A carrier oil is a neutral oil that *carries* the essential oil across your skin, thus diluting it and providing the right amount of healing oil. Examples of carrier oils are grapeseed, sweet almond, and jojoba oils.

You can find dilution calculators online to help establish the right amount of pure essential oil per product. Using the 2% rule, it approximately equals the following: for every 5 milliliters of carrier oil, use 1 to 2 drops of essential oil; for every 30 ml of carrier oil, use 12 drops of essential oil; and so on.

Essential oils are the preferred method to scent a natural product. They smell amazing and enhance any balm or cream. Although they have many healing benefits, as with anything, they have a list of warnings too. Please read and understand the warnings before you begin making your creations.

Warning

Never apply an essential oil directly to the skin. Always blend it with a carrier oil.

Citrus oils can make your skin photosensitive (extra-sensitive to the sun and more susceptible to sunburn). Therefore, avoid adding citrus essential oils to face creams and lip balms.

Use caution if pregnant or nursing, as some oils can be harmful. Ask your doctor first.

Always keep away from small children and pets.

Some essential oils are toxic to pets in particular. For dogs and cats, avoid tea tree, cinnamon, citrus, pine, sweet birch, wintergreen, and ylang ylang.

Here is a handy list of the most common oils and their uses. You can choose which oils to use in your DIY products.

Oil	Scent	Benefits	Mood
Bergamot	Lightly citrus	Good for acne, skin problems	Refreshing
Eucalyptus	Menthol	Anti-inflammatory	Clear
Lavender	Floral	Good for stress	Relaxing
Lemon	Citrus	Good for acne, skin problems	Refreshing
Orange	Fresh citrus	Combats fatigue, acne, depression	Uplifting
Peppermint	Minty	Combats fatigue, headaches	Awakening
Rose	Lightly floral	Good for skin, inflammation	Confident
Tea tree	Strong, menthol-like	Antibacterial, disinfectant Good for colds, congestion	Clean
Ylang ylang	Floral	Aphrodisiac	Sensual

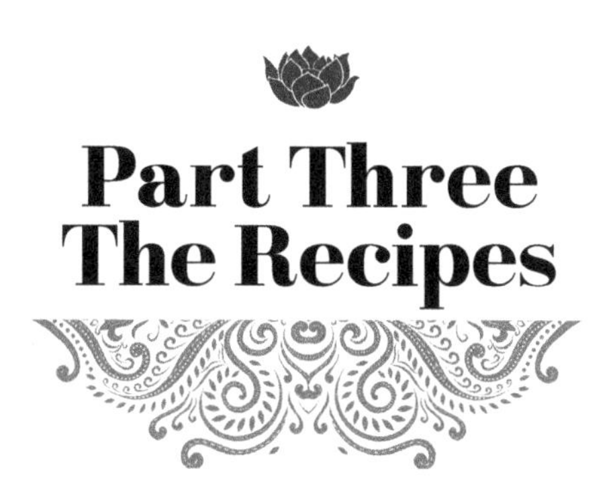

Part Three
The Recipes

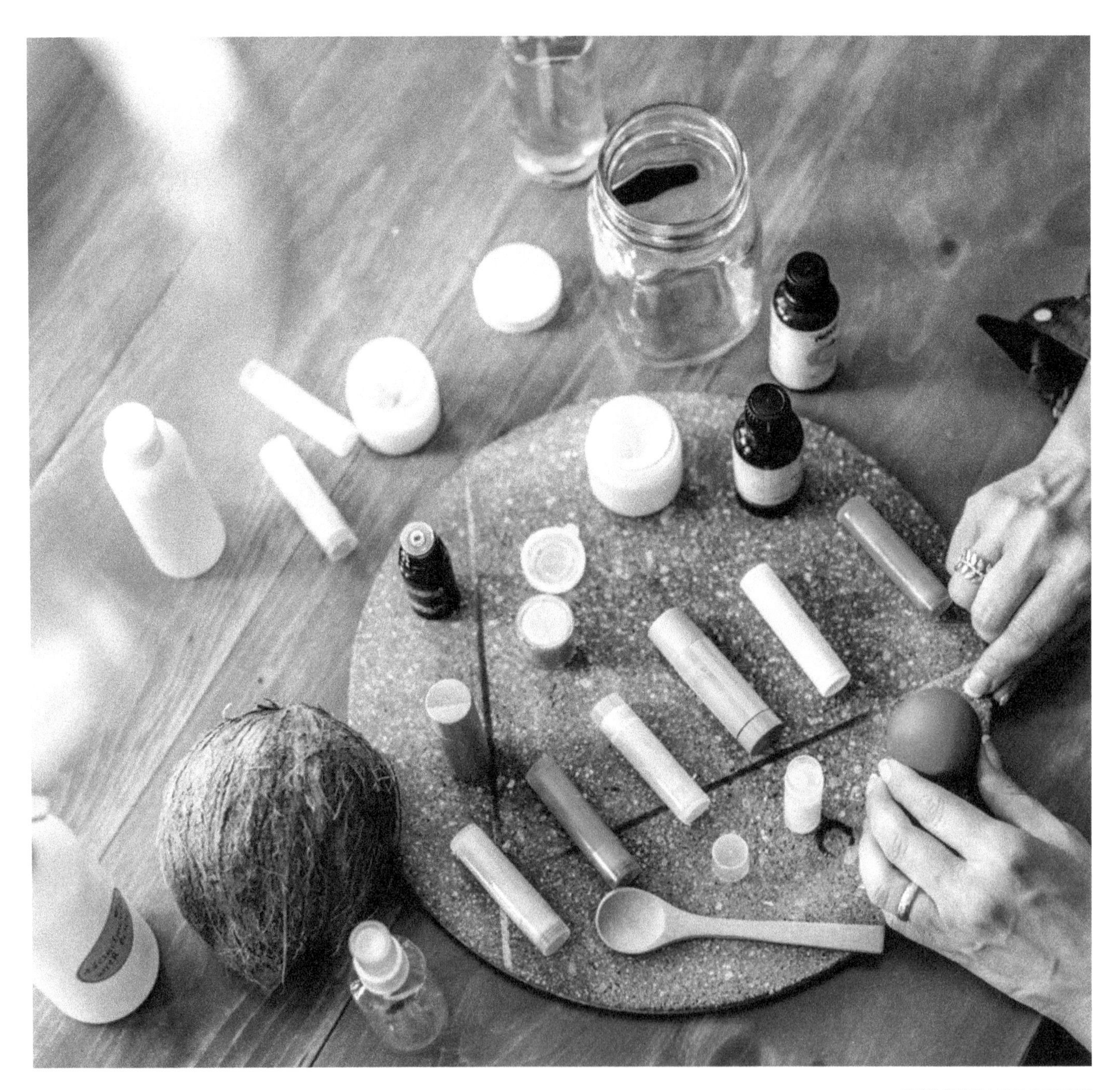

PHOTO CREDIT: **NAT CARON**

LIP BALM BASICS
Easy Step-by-Step Instructions

Lip balm is great for dry, chapped lips, and protective to sun rays and cold weather. What would we do without it? I personally can't go to sleep without applying lip balm first!

Do you have a preferred brand? I have analyzed today's most popular brands and what I've discovered is they are over-priced and contain fragrances and dyes that aren't healthy for our bodies.

Lip balm is cheap and easy to make, so why not just DIY?

If you follow my tutorials, you will soon be enjoying brand-name-style balms for a fraction of the price *and* it will be all-natural!

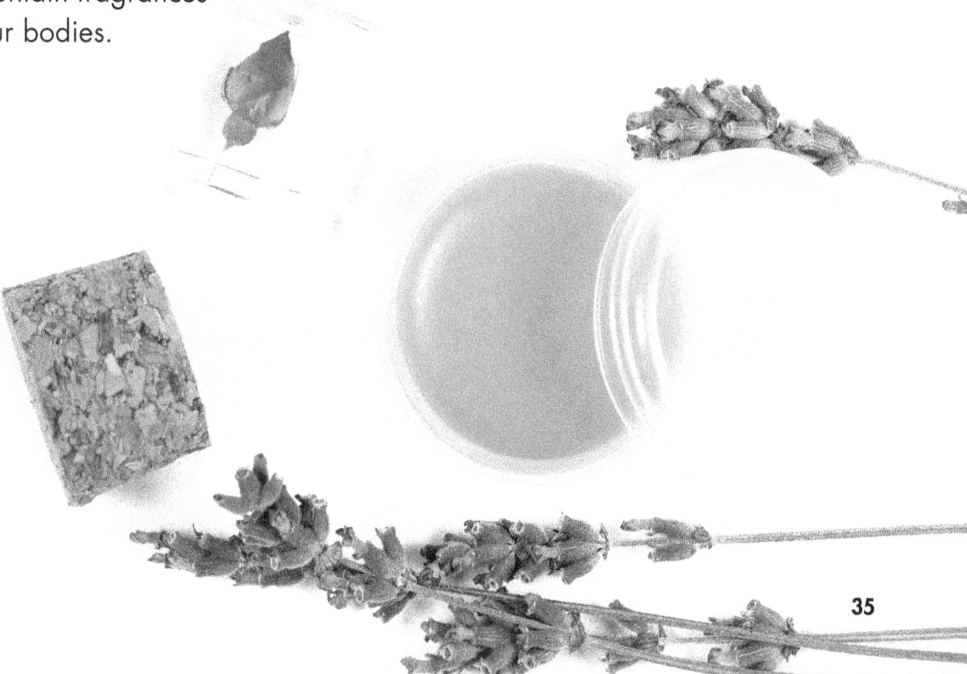

All-purpose lip balm

Inspired by your favourite store-bought brands

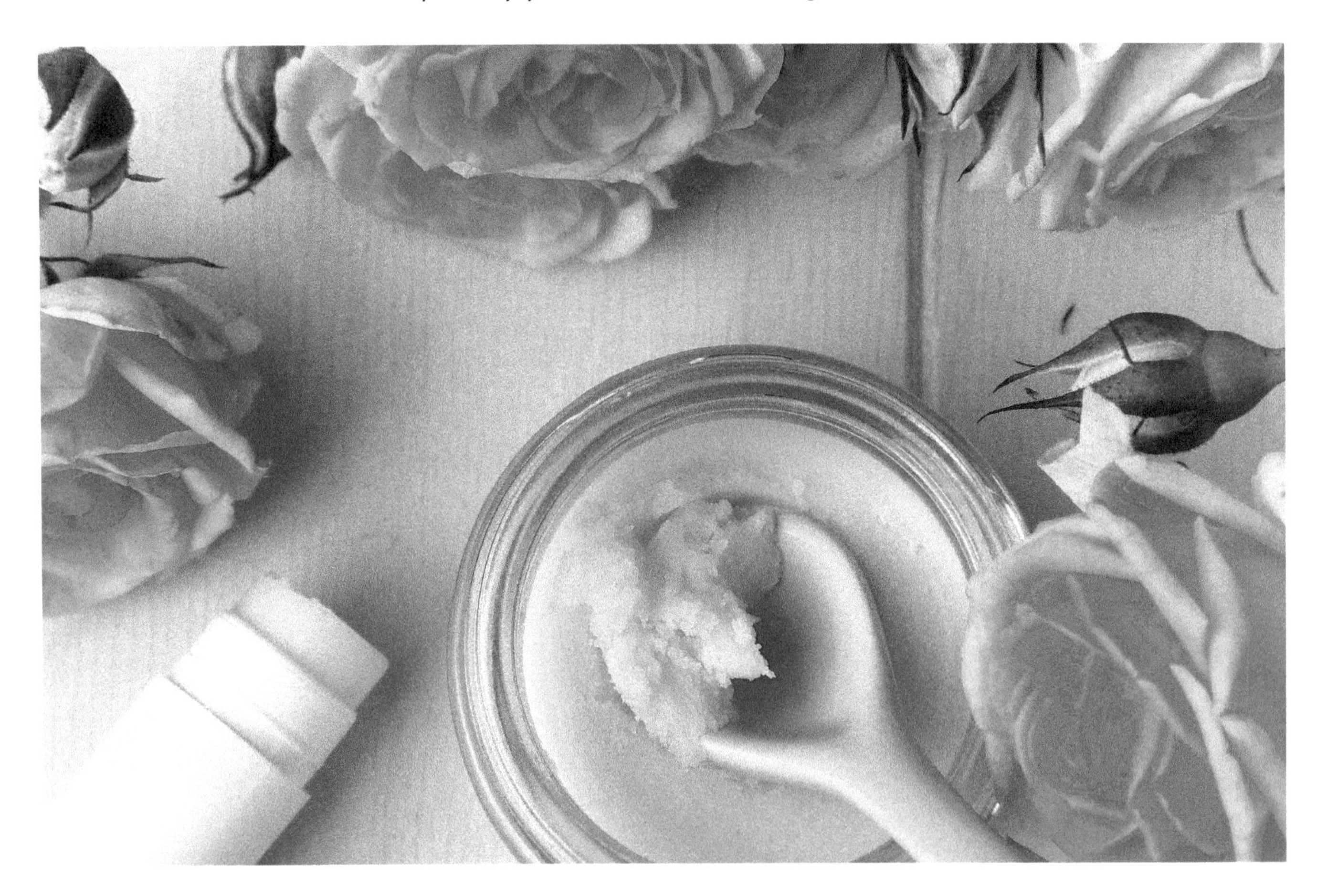

This is my go-to year-round lip balm recipe. It's a bit firmer and waxier, so I recommend it as a weather barrier and to soothe dry, chapped lips.

(Makes about 12 lip balms)

Equipment list

- Glass measuring cup
- 12 empty lip balm tubes or small round containers

Ingredients

- ¼ cup organic coconut oil (semi-hard type)
- ¼ cup shea butter
- ¼ cup + 2 tsp beeswax

Optional additions

- ½ tsp liquid stevia or flavoured stevia
- 10 drops of your favourite essential oil)
- ½ tsp food-grade clear extracts (e.g., peppermint, almond)

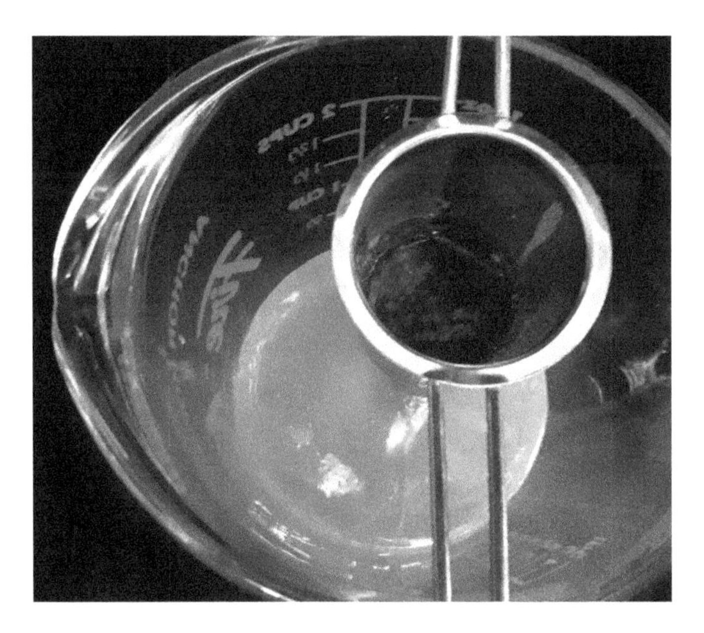

Instructions

Before beginning either method, be sure to remove the lip balm tube lids and set aside. Twist the tube mechanism to ensure it's working and set all the way to the bottom.

For the microwave

1. Measure out the coconut oil and shea butter, and put into the glass measuring cup. Microwave for 45 seconds. Remove and stir. Be careful as it will be very hot. Return to the microwave for 45 more seconds.
2. Once the oils begin to liquefy (but not boil), you can add the beeswax. Microwave for 30 seconds. Remove and stir. Continue heating in 30-second intervals until all of the beeswax has liquefied.
3. Stir in any optional additions, and carefully pour the liquid into the balm tubes. You can fill almost to the top. Try not to overpour, but if you do, it's easy to clean up later.

For the stove top

1. Fill a medium-sized clean pot with 3 to 4 cups water. Set on the stove burner, and place your glass measuring cup in the pot of water.
2. Measure out the coconut oil, shea butter, and beeswax. Put into the glass measuring cup, not into the water.
3. Turn on the stove to medium-low heat. This method heats slowly and does not scorch the ingredients. Stir constantly with a metal spoon, and never leave the oils unattended. Do not let the mixture boil.
4. Once your mixture is completely melted (about 15 minutes), turn off the stove and carefully remove the glass cup from the pot of water.
5. Stir in any optional additions, and carefully pour the liquid into the balm tubes. You can fill almost to the top. Try not to overpour, but if you do, it's easy to clean up later.

Tips

We don't recommend citrus essential oils for lip balm, as citrus makes the skin photosensitive and can result in sunburns.

The balms will begin to harden immediately, so work quickly.

If the liquid in the measuring cup begins to harden, simply microwave it again for 25 seconds and stir.

You may find, as the balms harden, there is an indentation or hole that appears in the wax. That is completely normal. If you prefer the look of a smooth finish, take the straight side of a butter knife and scrape it across the balm.

Chocolate Mint Lip Balm

Satisfy your craving

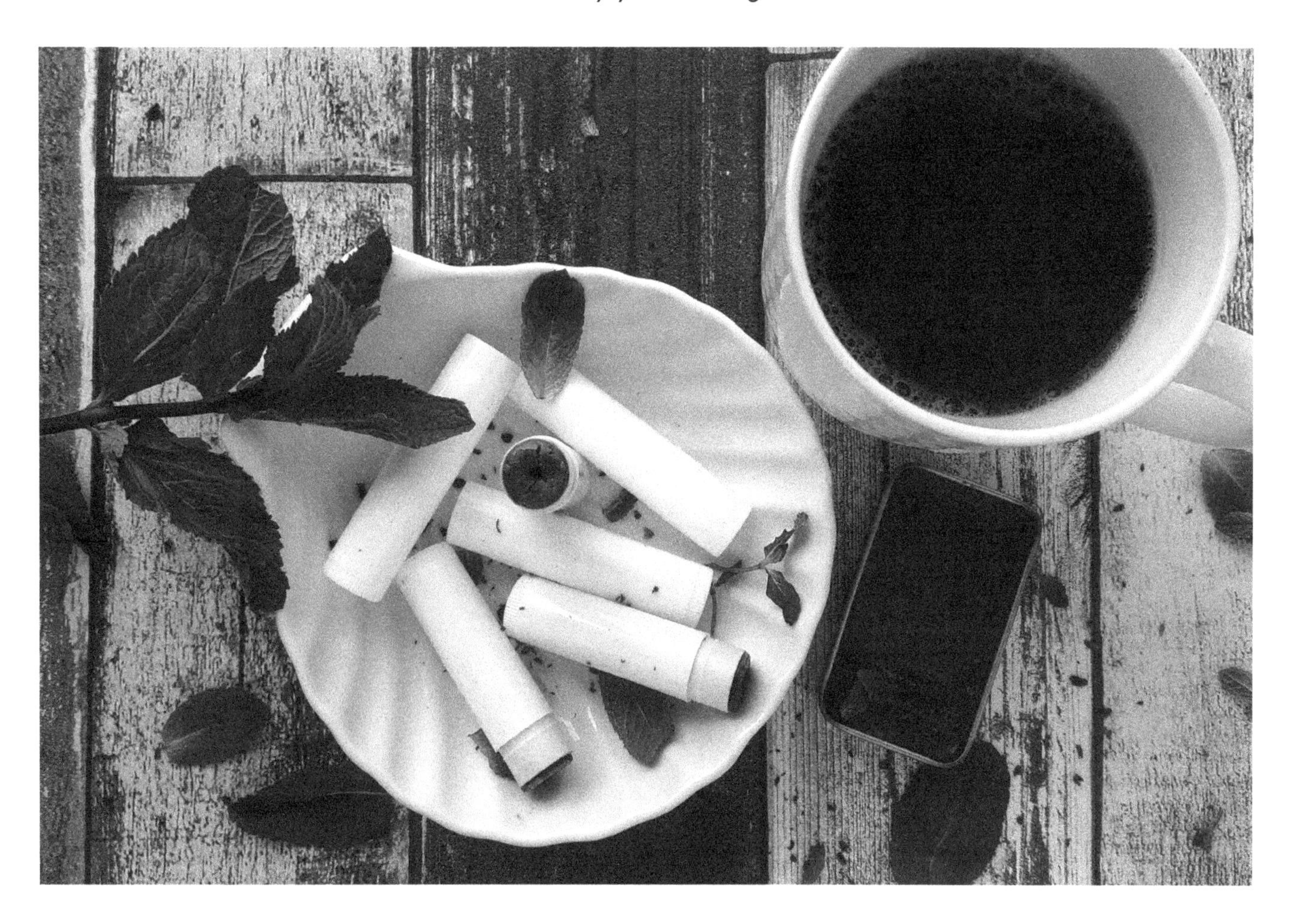

If you're like me, a chocoholic, you will find the scent of this lip balm very satisfying to the senses.

(Makes about 12 lip balms)

Equipment list

- Glass measuring cup
- 12 empty lip balm tubes or small round containers

Optional additions

- ½ tsp liquid stevia or chocolate-flavoured stevia
- 1 tsp organic cocoa powder
- ¼ tsp pure peppermint extract or 15 drops peppermint essential oil

Ingredients

- ¼ cup organic coconut oil (semi-hard)
- ¼ cup shea butter
- ¼ cup beeswax

Instructions

Before beginning either method, be sure to remove the lip balm tube lids and set aside. Twist the tube mechanism to ensure it's working and set all the way to the bottom.

For the microwave

1. Measure out the coconut oil and shea butter, and put into the glass measuring cup. Microwave for 45 seconds. Remove and stir. Be careful as it will be very hot. Return to the microwave for 45 more seconds.
2. Once the oils begin to liquefy (but not boil), you can add the beeswax. Microwave for 30 seconds. Remove and stir. Continue heating in 30-second intervals until all of the beeswax has liquefied.
3. Stir in any optional additions, and carefully pour the liquid into the balm tubes. You can fill almost to the top. Try not to overpour, but if you do, it's easy to clean up later.

For the stove top

1. Fill a medium-sized clean pot with 3 to 4 cups water. Set on the stove burner, and place your glass measuring cup in the pot of water.
2. Measure out the coconut oil, shea butter, and beeswax. Put into the glass measuring cup, not into the water.
3. Turn on the stove to medium-low heat. This method heats slowly and does not scorch the ingredients. Stir constantly with a metal spoon, and never leave the oils unattended. Do not let the mixture boil.
4. Once your mixture is completely melted (about 15 minutes), turn off the stove and carefully remove the glass cup from the pot of water.

5. Stir in any optional additions, and carefully pour the liquid into the balm tubes. You can fill almost to the top. Try not to overpour, but if you do, it is easy to clean up later.

Tips

Always mix powder with the cold coconut oil first. If you add the powder to the melted oils, it may clump your balm.

The balms will begin to harden immediately, so work quickly.

If the liquid in the measuring cup begins to harden, simply microwave it again for 25 seconds and stir.

You may find, as the balms harden, there is an indentation or hole that appears in the wax. That is completely normal. If you prefer the look of a smooth finish, take the straight side of a butter knife and scrape it across the balm.

Rose Lip Balm

Fresh and floral

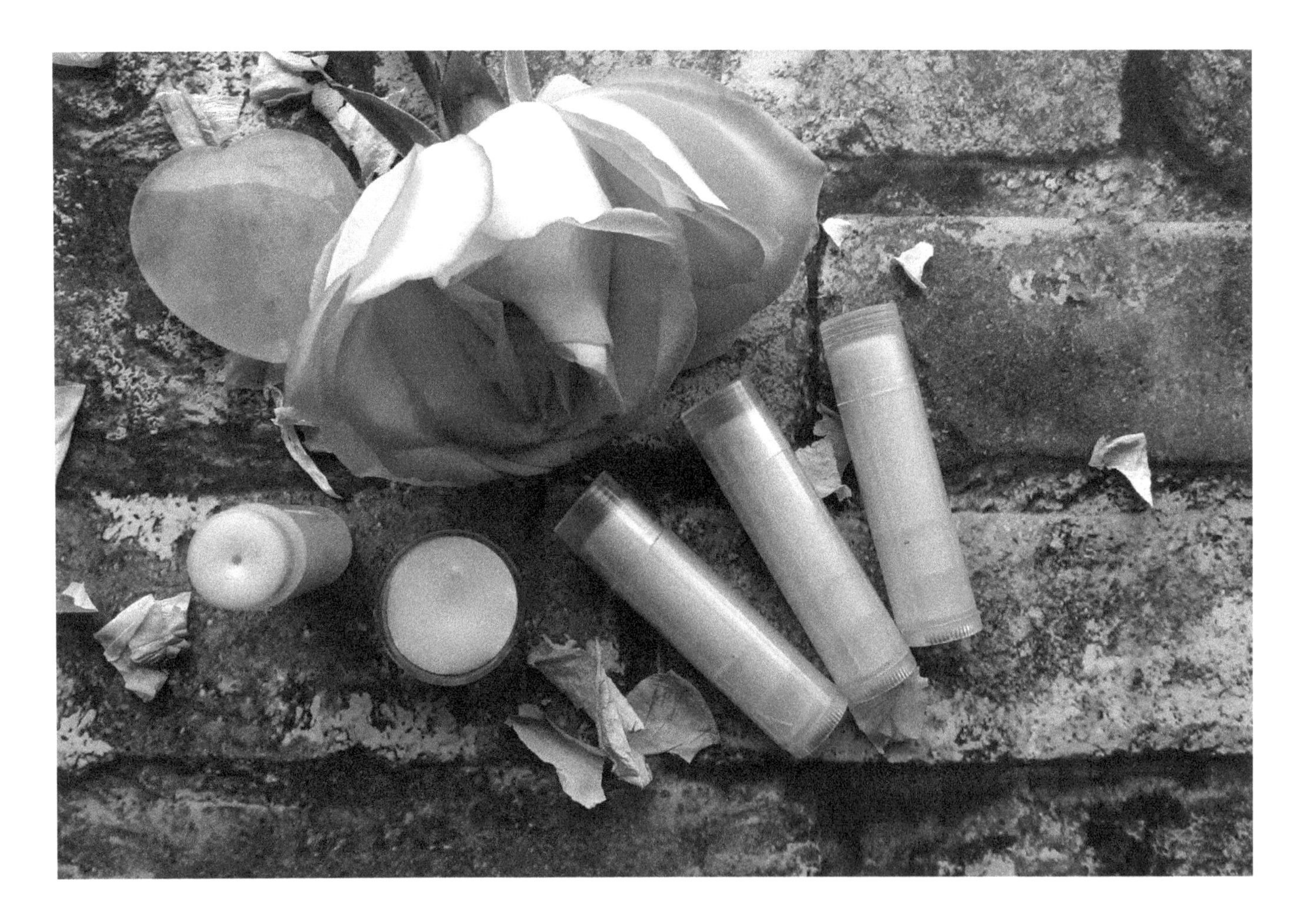

Enjoy the sweet smell of roses. Light and feminine, and a beneficial essential oil for the skin.

(Makes about 12 lip balms)

Equipment list

- Glass measuring cup
- 12 empty lip balm tubes or small round containers

Optional additions

- ½ tsp liquid stevia
- 1 tsp hibiscus powder or beetroot powder
- 25 drops rose essential oil

Ingredients

- ¼ cup organic coconut oil (semi-hard)
- ¼ cup shea butter
- ¼ cup beeswax

Instructions

Before beginning either method, be sure to remove the lip balm tube lids and set aside. Twist the tube mechanism to ensure it's working and set all the way to the bottom.

For the microwave

1. Measure out the coconut oil and shea butter, and put into the glass measuring cup. Microwave for 45 seconds. Remove and stir. Be careful as it will be very hot. Return to the microwave for 45 more seconds.
2. Once the oils begin to liquefy (but not boil), you can add the beeswax. Microwave for 30 seconds. Remove and stir. Continue heating in 30-second intervals until all of the beeswax has liquefied.
3. Stir in any optional additions, and carefully pour the liquid into the balm tubes. You can fill almost to the top. Try not to overpour, but if you do, it's easy to clean up later.

For the stove top

1. Fill a medium-sized clean pot with 3 to 4 cups water. Set on the stove burner, and place your glass measuring cup in the pot of water.
2. Measure out the coconut oil, shea butter, and beeswax. Put into the glass measuring cup, <u>not</u> into the water.
3. Turn on the stove to medium-low heat. This method heats slowly and does not scorch the ingredients. Stir constantly with a metal spoon, and never leave the oils unattended. Do not let the mixture boil.
4. Once your mixture is completely melted (about 15 minutes), turn off the stove and carefully remove the glass cup from the pot of water.

5. Stir in any optional additions, and carefully pour the liquid into the balm tubes. You can fill almost to the top. Try not to overpour, but if you do, it's easy to clean up later.

Tips

Always mix powder with the cold coconut oil first. If you add the powder to the melted oils, it may clump your balm.

If the melted liquid seems clumpy, due to the hibiscus or beetroot powder, strain the melted liquid through a fine tea strainer into a second glass container. This will catch any overcooked powder, leaving a smoother liquid.

The balms will begin to harden immediately, so work quickly.

If the liquid in the measuring cup begins to harden, simply microwave it again for 25 seconds and stir.

You may find, as the balms harden, there is an indentation or hole that appears in the wax. That is completely normal. If you prefer the look of a smooth finish, take the straight side of a butter knife and scrape it across the balm.

Moisturizing Lip Balm Ball

Comparable to EOS lip balm

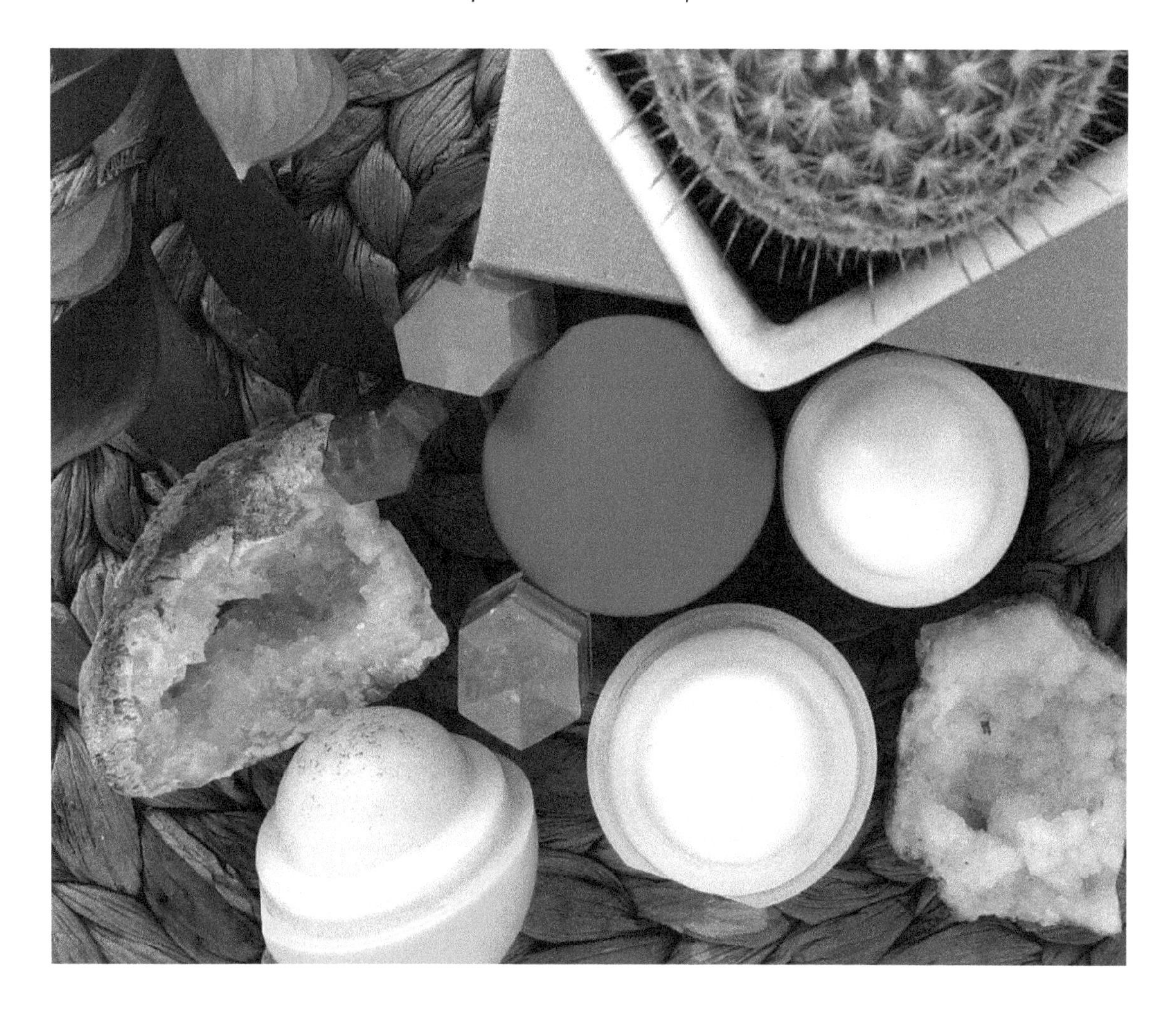

A fun lip balm container and a soft moisturizing texture at a fraction of the store price.

(Makes about 6 lip balms)

Equipment list

- Glass measuring cup
- 6 empty lip balm balls (3 parts)

Ingredients

- ¼ cup coconut oil (semi-hard)
- ¼ cup shea butter
- ¼ cup beeswax
- 1 tsp vitamin E oil

Optional additions

- ½ tsp liquid stevia or flavoured stevia
- 20 drops of your favourite essential oil
- ¼ tsp food-grade clear extracts

Instructions

Before you begin, you'll need to assemble the ball tube. Remove the lid and set aside. Remove the mesh piece and screw it into the lid. You will be filling to the top of the coloured piece. (See photo.)

For the microwave

1. Measure out the coconut oil and shea butter, and put into the glass measuring cup. Microwave for 45 seconds. Remove and stir. Be careful as it will be very hot. Return to the microwave for 45 more seconds.
2. Once the oils begin to liquefy (but not boil), you can add the beeswax. Microwave for 30 seconds. Remove and stir. Continue heating in 30-second intervals until all of the beeswax has liquefied.
3. Stir in vitamin E and any optional additions, and carefully pour the liquid into the balm balls. You can fill almost to the top. Try not to overpour, but if you do, it's easy to clean up later.

For the stove top

1. Fill a medium-sized clean pot with 3 to 4 cups water. Set on the stove burner, and place your glass measuring cup in the pot of water.
2. Measure out the coconut oil, shea butter, and beeswax. Put into the glass measuring cup, not into the water.
3. Turn on the stove to medium-low heat. This method heats slowly and does not scorch the ingredients. Stir constantly with a metal spoon, and never leave the oils unattended. Do not let the mixture boil.
4. Once your mixture is completely melted (about 15 minutes), turn off the stove and carefully remove the glass cup from the pot of water.
5. Stir in vitamin E and any optional additions, and carefully pour the liquid into the balm balls. You can fill almost to the top. Try not to overpour, but if you do, it's easy to clean up later.

Tips

The balms will begin to harden immediately, so work quickly.

If the liquid in the measuring cup begins to harden, simply microwave it again for 25 seconds and stir.

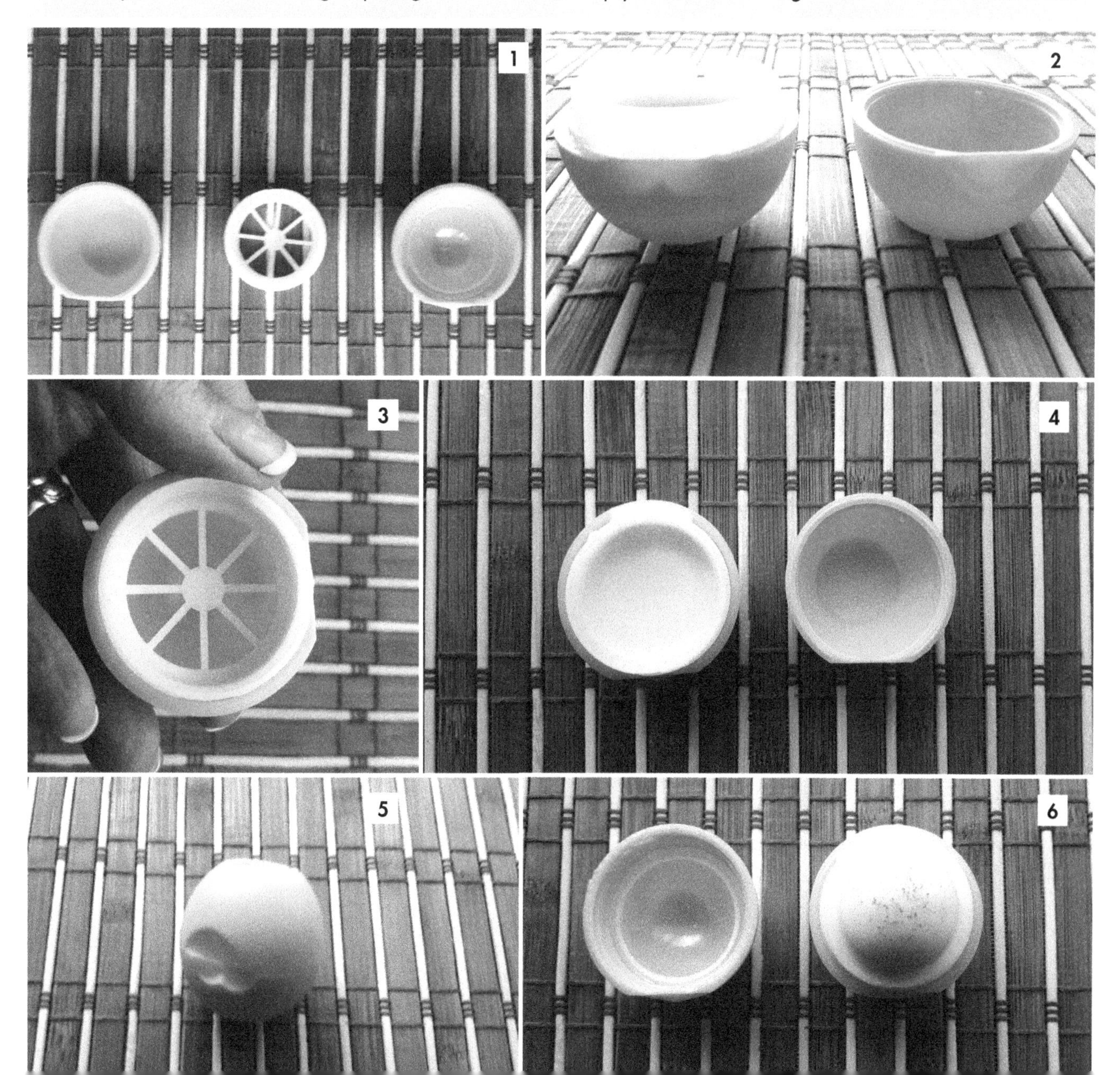

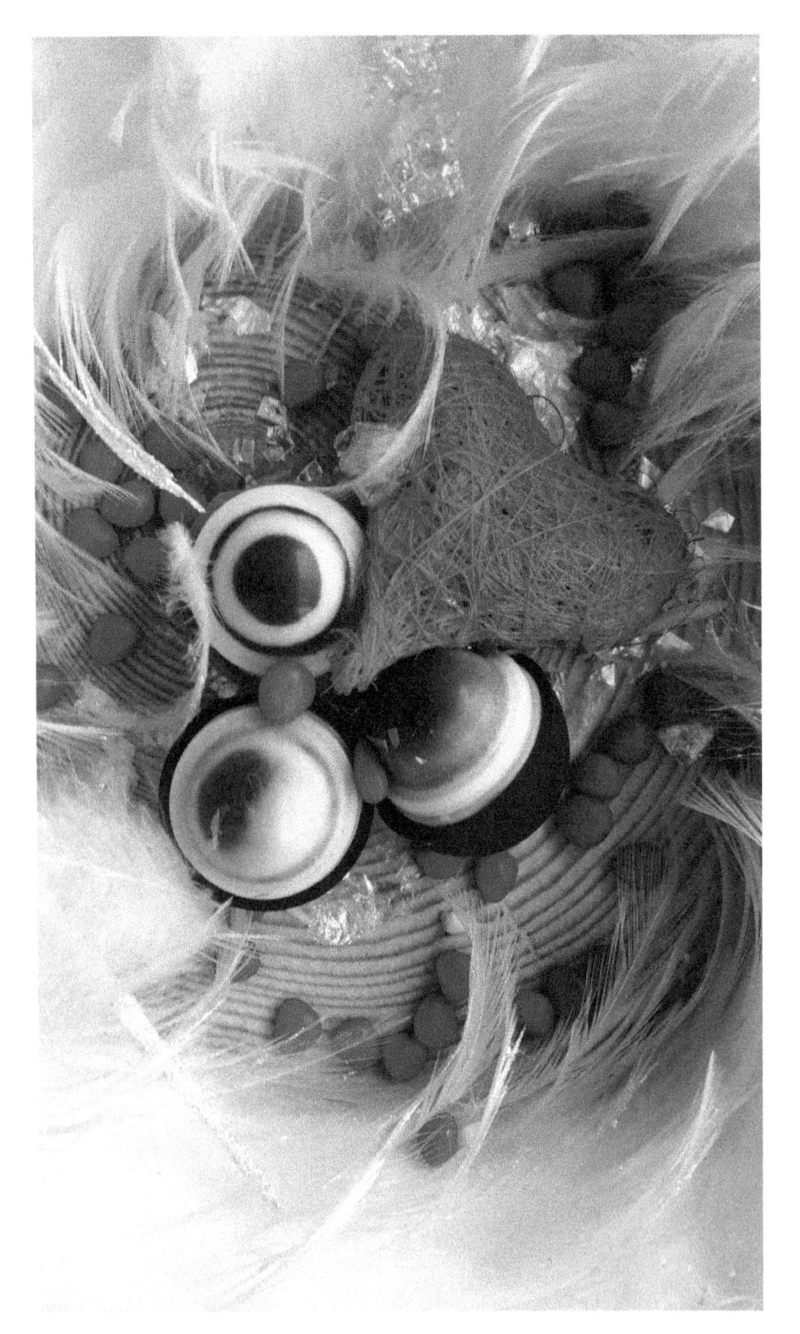

Vanilla-Chocolate Striped Balm

The best of both flavours

This recipe is a bit more challenging because you work with two flavours of balm at the same time, alternating between the two flavours as you pour them to create stripes. If you have patience, the result is worth it!

(Makes about 6 lip balms)

Equipment list

- 2 glass measuring cups
- 6 empty lip balm balls (3 parts)
- Small baking tray

Ingredients

- ¼ cup coconut oil (semi-firm)
- ¼ cup shea butter
- ¼ cup beeswax
- ¼ tsp cocoa powder
- ½ tsp liquid vanilla stevia

Instructions

- Before you begin, you'll need to assemble the sphere tube. Remove the lid and set aside. Remove the mesh piece and screw it into the lid. You will be filling to the top of the coloured piece (see photo.)
- Assemble the prepared balm ball on a small baking tray.

For the microwave

1. Measure out the coconut oil and shea butter, and put into the first glass measuring cup. Microwave for 45 seconds. Remove and stir. Be careful as it will be very hot. Return to the microwave for 45 more seconds.
2. Once the oils begin to liquefy (but not boil), you can add the beeswax. Microwave for 30 seconds. Remove and stir. Continue heating in 30-second intervals until all of the beeswax has liquefied.
3. Stir in any optional additions, and carefully pour the liquid into the balm balls. You can fill almost to the top. Try not to overpour, but if you do, it's easy to clean up later.
4. Pour half the liquid into the second glass measuring cup.
5. Stir cocoa powder into the first glass cup and vanilla stevia into the second glass cup.
6. Pour a small amount of chocolate or vanilla balm into the bottom of the ball.
7. Place the baking tray in the fridge for 5 minutes, and then pour a layer of the other balm colour.
8. Return to the fridge for 5 minutes.
9. Fill your last layer to cover the plastic middle piece of the sphere mold. Chill in the fridge for 30 minutes. Pop on the bottom portion of the container and twist off. You should have a lovely round stripy lip balm.

For the stove top

1. Fill a medium-sized clean pot with 3 to 4 cups water. Set on the stove burner, and place your first glass measuring cup in the pot of water.
2. Measure out the coconut oil, shea butter, and beeswax. Put into the glass measuring cup, <u>not</u> into the water.
3. Turn on the stove to medium-low heat. This method heats slowly and does not scorch the ingredients. Stir constantly with a metal spoon, and never leave the oils unattended. Do not let the mixture boil.
4. Once your mixture is completely melted (about 15 minutes), turn off the stove and carefully remove the glass cup from the pot of water.
5. Pour half the liquid into the second glass measuring cup.

6. Stir cocoa powder into the first glass cup and vanilla stevia into the second glass cup.
7. Pour a small amount of chocolate or vanilla balm into the bottom of the ball.
8. Place the baking tray in the fridge for 5 minutes, and then pour a layer of the other balm colour.
9. Return to the fridge for 5 minutes.
10. Fill your last layer to cover the plastic middle piece of the sphere mould. Chill in the fridge for 30 minutes. Pop on the bottom portion of the container and twist off. You should have a lovely round stripy lip balm.

Tips

Resist the temptation to open up the balm tubes early. Wait the full 30 minutes.

The liquid in the measuring cup will begin to harden, so you'll need to reheat it a few times throughout the process.

If your lip ball does not set correctly due to inadequate chilling time, put it back in the fridge for another 20 minutes. This usually resolves it.

For a quicker version of this recipe, pour the alternating lip balms over one another at once and then chill for 30 minutes. The result is a marble effect.

Matcha Green Tea Balm

Rich and earthy

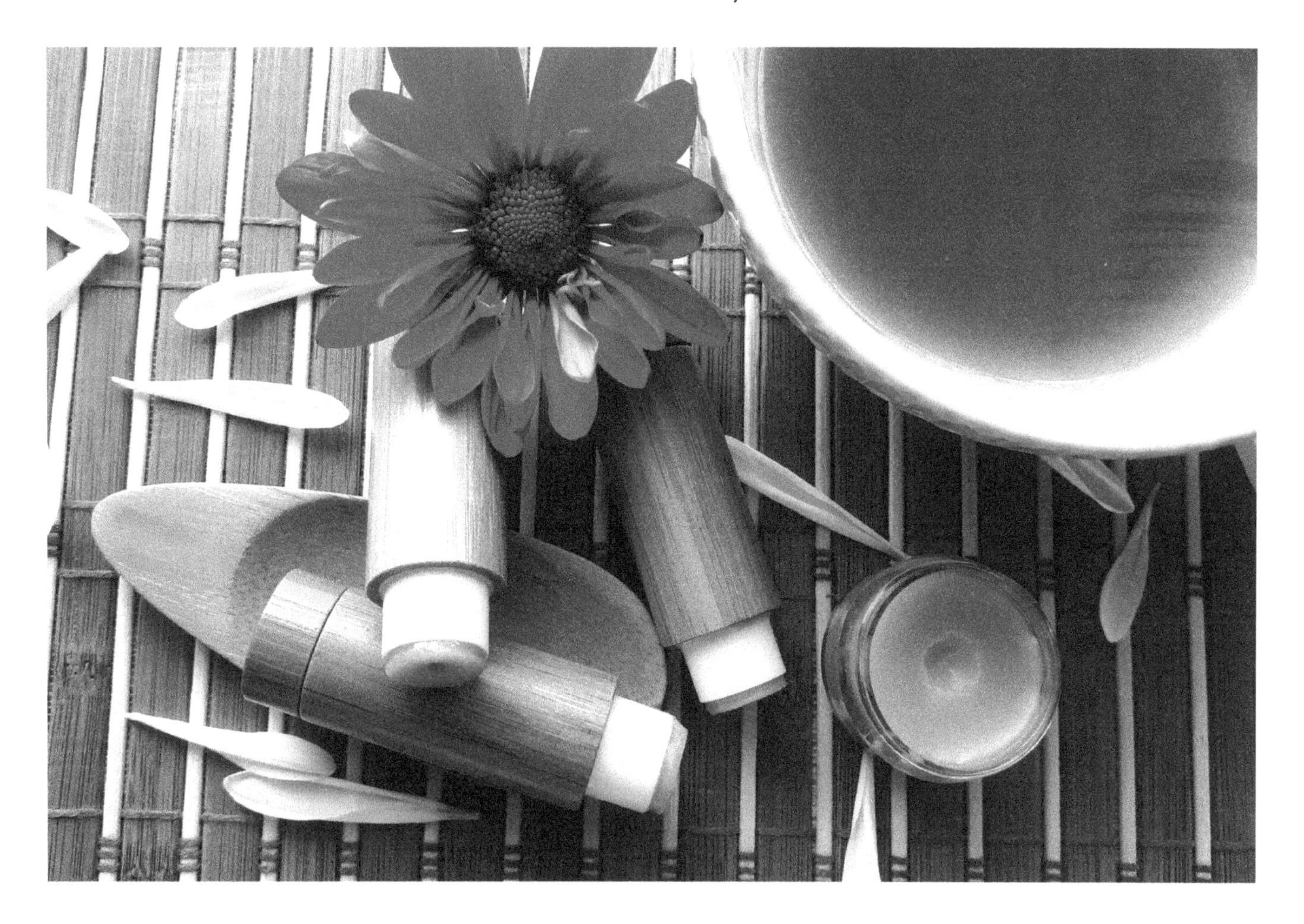

Green tea balm is another favourite due to the colour and earthy aroma. It's full of antioxidants, which are great for your skin!

(Makes about 12 lip balms)

Equipment list

- Glass measuring cup
- 12 empty lip balm tubes or small round containers

Ingredients

- ¼ cup coconut oil (semi-hard)
- ¼ cup shea butter
- ¼ cup beeswax
- ¼ tsp vitamin E oil
- ¼ tsp vanilla stevia
- 1 tsp matcha tea powder

Instructions

Before beginning either method, be sure to remove the lip balm tube lids and set aside. Twist the tube mechanism to ensure it's working and set all the way to the bottom.

For the microwave

1. Measure out the coconut oil and shea butter, and put into the glass measuring cup. Microwave for 45 seconds. Remove and stir. Be careful as it will be very hot. Return to the microwave for 45 more seconds.
2. Once the oils begin to liquefy (but not boil), you can add the beeswax. Microwave for 30 seconds. Remove and stir. Continue heating in 30-second intervals until all of the beeswax has liquefied.
3. Stir in the matcha tea powder and carefully pour the liquid into the balm tubes. You can fill almost to the top. Try not to overpour, but if you do, it's easy to clean up later.

For the stove top

1. Fill a medium-sized clean pot with 3 to 4 cups water. Set on the stove burner, and place your glass measuring cup in the pot of water.
2. Measure out the coconut oil, shea butter, and beeswax. Put into the glass measuring cup, not into the water.
3. Turn on the stove to medium-low heat. This method heats slowly and does not scorch the ingredients. Stir constantly with a metal spoon, and never leave the oils unattended. Do not let the mixture boil.
4. Once your mixture is completely melted (about 15 minutes), turn off the stove and carefully remove the glass cup from the pot of water.

5. Stir in the rest of the ingredients, and carefully pour the liquid into the balm tubes. You can fill almost to the top. Try not to overpour, but if you do, it's easy to clean up later.

Tips

Always mix powder with the cold coconut oil first. If you add the powder to the melted oils, it may clump your balm.

The balms will begin to harden immediately, so work quickly.

If the liquid in the measuring cup begins to harden, simply microwave it again for 25 seconds and stir.

You may find, as the balms harden, there is an indentation or hole that appears in the wax. That is completely normal. If you prefer the look of a smooth finish, take the straight side of a butter knife and scrape it across the balm.

Candy Cane Lip Balm

Fun and festive

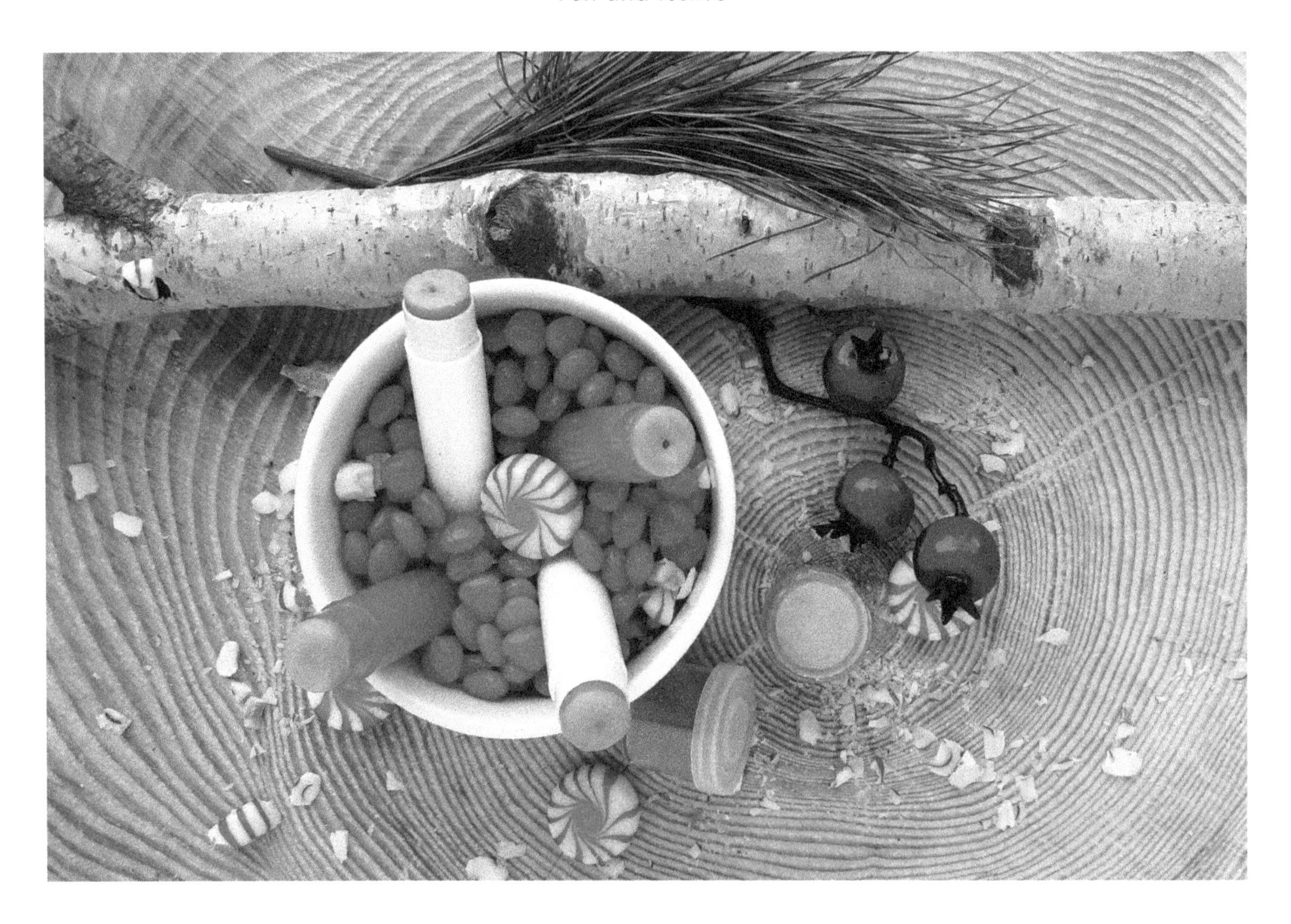

This is a fun and festive lip balm, which can double as cinnamon hearts around Valentine's Day. Smells and tastes great, plus the cinnamon can give you a lip-plumping effect.

(Makes about 12 lip balms)

Equipment list

- Glass measuring cup
- 12 empty lip balm tubes or small round containers

Ingredients

- ¼ cup coconut oil (semi-hard)
- ¼ cup shea butter
- ¼ cup beeswax
- ¼ tsp stevia
- 1 tsp hibiscus powder or beetroot powder
- ½ tsp real peppermint extract or 15 drops peppermint essential oil
- 15 drops cinnamon bark essential oil

Instructions

Before beginning either method, be sure to remove the lip balm tube lids and set aside. Twist the tube mechanism to ensure it's working and set all the way to the bottom.

For the microwave

1. Measure out the coconut oil and shea butter, and put into the glass measuring cup. Microwave for 45 seconds. Remove and stir. Be careful as it will be very hot. Return to the microwave for 45 more seconds.
2. Once the oils begin to liquefy (but not boil), you can add the beeswax. Microwave for 30 seconds. Remove and stir. Continue heating in 30-second intervals until all of the beeswax has liquefied.
3. Carefully pour the liquid into the balm tubes. You can fill almost to the top. Try not to overpour, but if you do, it's easy to clean up later.

For the stove top

1. Fill a medium-sized clean pot with 3 to 4 cups water. Set on the stove burner, and place your glass measuring cup in the pot of water.
2. Measure out the coconut oil, shea butter, and beeswax. Put into the glass measuring cup, <u>not</u> into the water.
3. Turn on the stove to medium-low heat. This method heats slowly and does not scorch the ingredients. Stir constantly with a metal spoon, and never leave the oils unattended. Do not let the mixture boil.

4. Once your mixture is completely melted (about 15 minutes), turn off the stove and carefully remove the glass cup from the pot of water.

5. Carefully pour the liquid into the balm tubes. You can fill almost to the top. Try not to overpour, but if you do, it's easy to clean up later.

Tips

Always mix powder with the cold coconut oil first. If you add the powder to the melted oils, it may clump your balm.

The balms will begin to harden immediately, so work quickly.

If the liquid in the measuring cup begins to harden, simply microwave it again for 25 seconds and stir.

You may find, as the balms harden, there is an indentation or hole that appears in the wax. That is completely normal. If you prefer the look of a smooth finish, take the straight side of a butter knife and scrape it across the balm.

BODY LOTION 101

Moisturizing Recipes

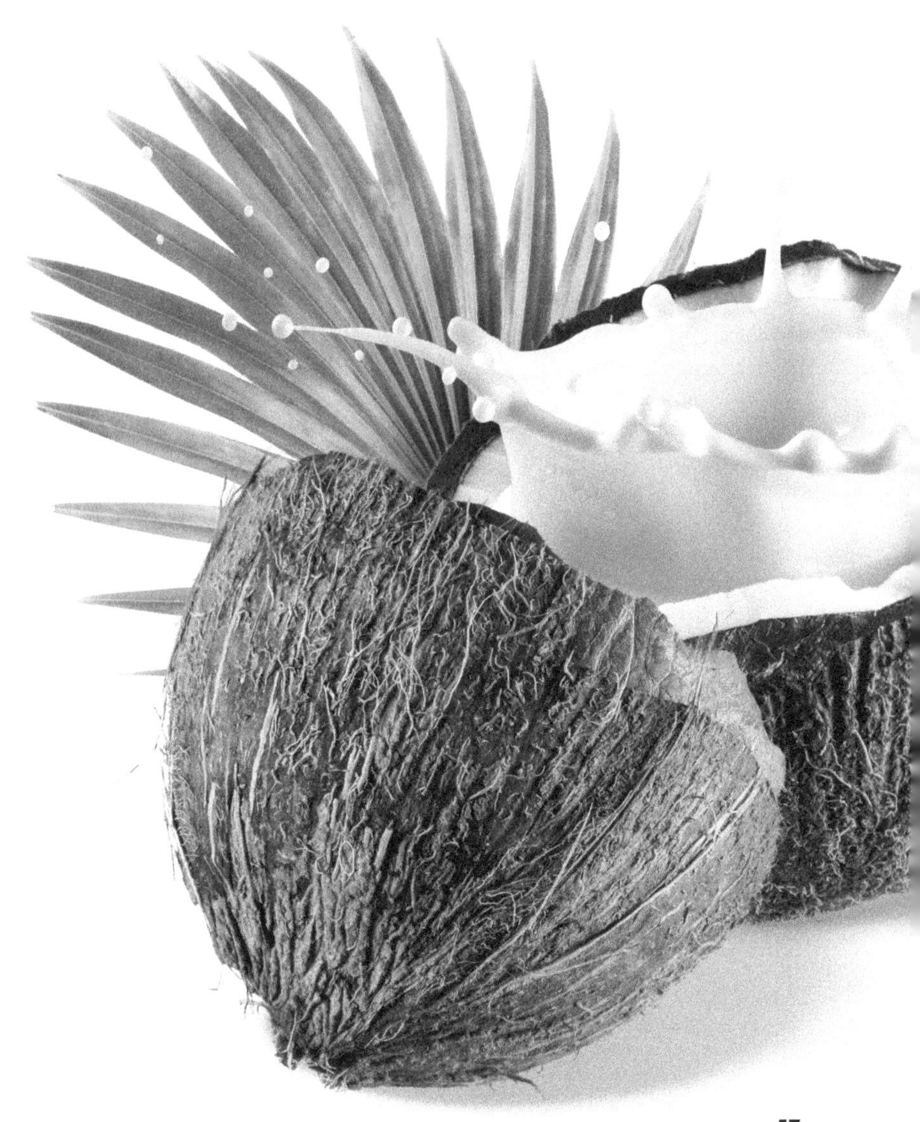

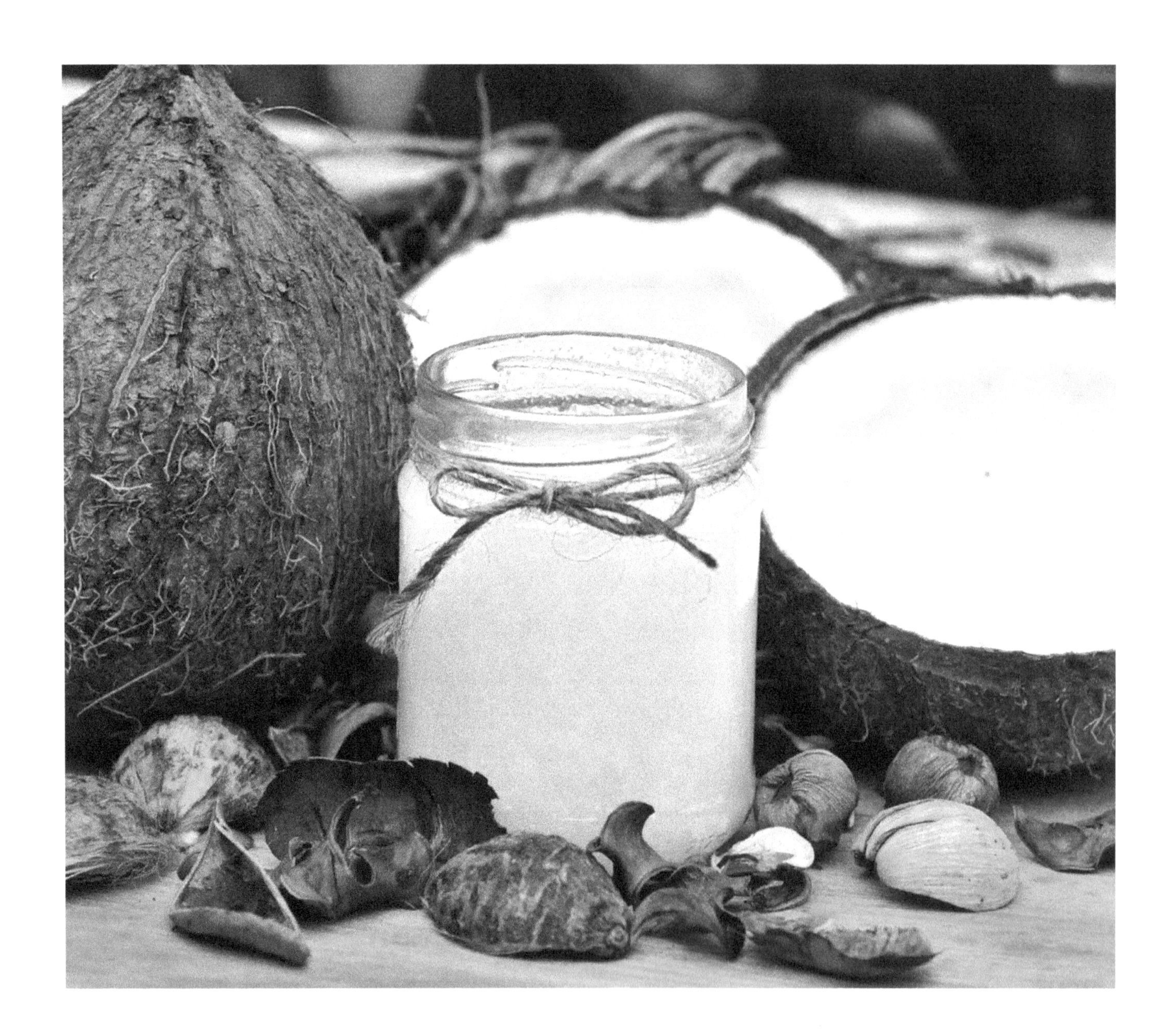

There are so many lotions on the shelves, each promising something new and improved. Do you buy a particular brand or just what's on sale? Ever look at the ingredients first? Many of us just buy what's priced best and go. I used to do that all the time until I realized the truth of what's really in our body products.

Did you know petroleum (also known as mineral oil) is a common ingredient in body lotions? According to the National Center for Biotechnology Information (NCBI) "mineral oil hydrocarbons are the greatest contaminant of the human body, amounting to approximately 1 g per person."[1] This is shocking as petroleum is found in so many of our products, including baby products. Studies also showed that nursing women who used petroleum-based products had this chemical in their breast milk.

Another study by the NCBI tested mice to see if tumour growth increased with the use of petroleum-based products twice a week for twenty weeks. The results: an increase in the rate of formation and number of tumours found where the cream was applied topically.

NCBI conducted a study in 2011 and found this: "The present study indicates that petroleum-based oils contain compounds with possible endocrine-disrupting potential, some of them acting via the hormone receptors."[2]

Did you know that body lotion doesn't cost a lot to make? What we're paying for is the label, the packaging, and the promise of beauty. The beauty industry is huge! And we're all buying into it – until now.

Popular body lotions contain artificial fragrance, petroleum, and other toxic chemicals. What if I told you, you could create your own body lotion that feels better on your skin, smells amazing, and is inexpensive? I'll teach you how to DIY your favourite body creams.

Here are my versions of a deeply hydrating body lotion and a cocoa butter body lotion.

Deeply Moisturizing Body Lotion

No petroleum here

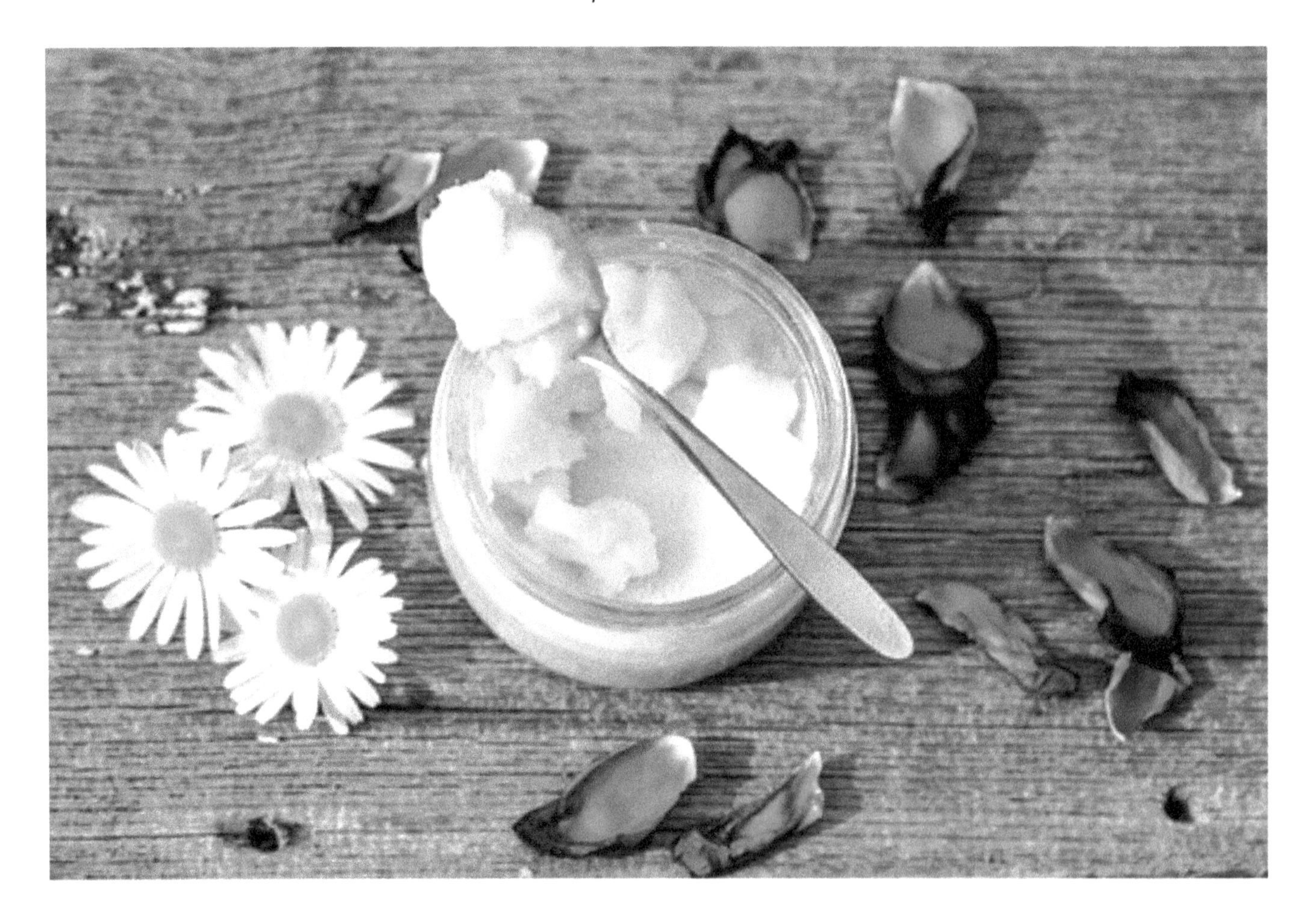

I recommend using this lotion on very dry skin or during the winter months. It may go on a bit greasy but absorbs quickly into the skin.

(Makes one small jar)

Equipment list

- Small mason jar or Boston jar with lid
- Food processor

Ingredients

- ½ cup avocado butter
- ½ cup coconut oil (semi-hard)
- 1 tsp vitamin E oil
- 10 drops of your favourite essential oil

Instructions

1. Measure out the avocado butter and coconut oil, and add to your food processor.
2. Mix for 1 minute. Pour in your vitamin E oil and essential oils while blending.
3. Scoop into clean, dry glass jars. It's ready for immediate use.
4. Store in a cool place.

Creamy Cocoa Butter Body Lotion

Smells amazing!

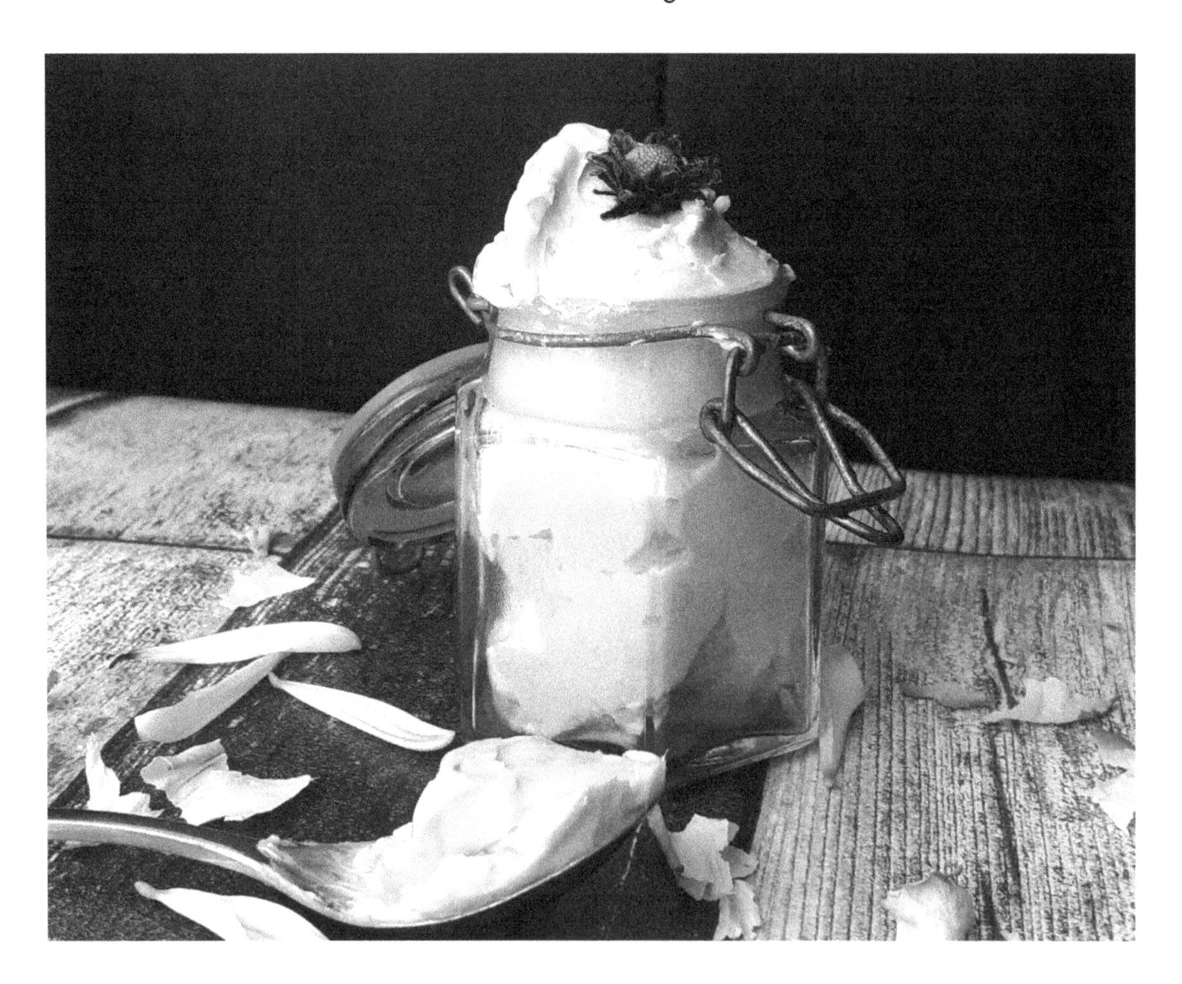

A perfect year-round moisturizer.
Beneficial in preventing stretch marks too!

(Makes one small jar)

Equipment list

- Glass measuring cup
- Small 8-oz jar with lid

Ingredients

- ¼ cup cocoa butter
- ¼ cup shea butter
- ¼ cup coconut oil (semi-hard)

Instructions

You can melt the butters in a microwave or on the stove top.

For the microwave

1. Measure out the butters and coconut oil, and add to the glass measuring cup.
2. Microwave for 45 seconds, stir, and microwave again for 30 seconds.
3. Continue microwaving in 30-second intervals until the mixture is completely melted.
4. Once melted, pour into clean, dry glass jars.
5. Let set for several hours or overnight. Store in a cool place.

For the stove top

1. Fill a medium-sized clean pot with 3 to 4 cups water. Place on the stove burner.
2. Measure out the butters and coconut oil, and add to the glass measuring cup.
3. Place your glass measuring cup in the pot of water.
4. Turn on the stove to medium-low setting. Turn the numbered dial to about four. This method heats slowly and does not scorch the ingredients.
5. With a metal spoon, stir constantly. Never leave the oils unattended.
6. Once your mixture is completely melted (about 15 minutes), turn off the stove and carefully remove the glass cup from the pot of water.
7. Fill your glass container, and let it set for several hours or overnight. Store in a cool place.

Vanilla-Lavender Body Whip

Heaven in a jar

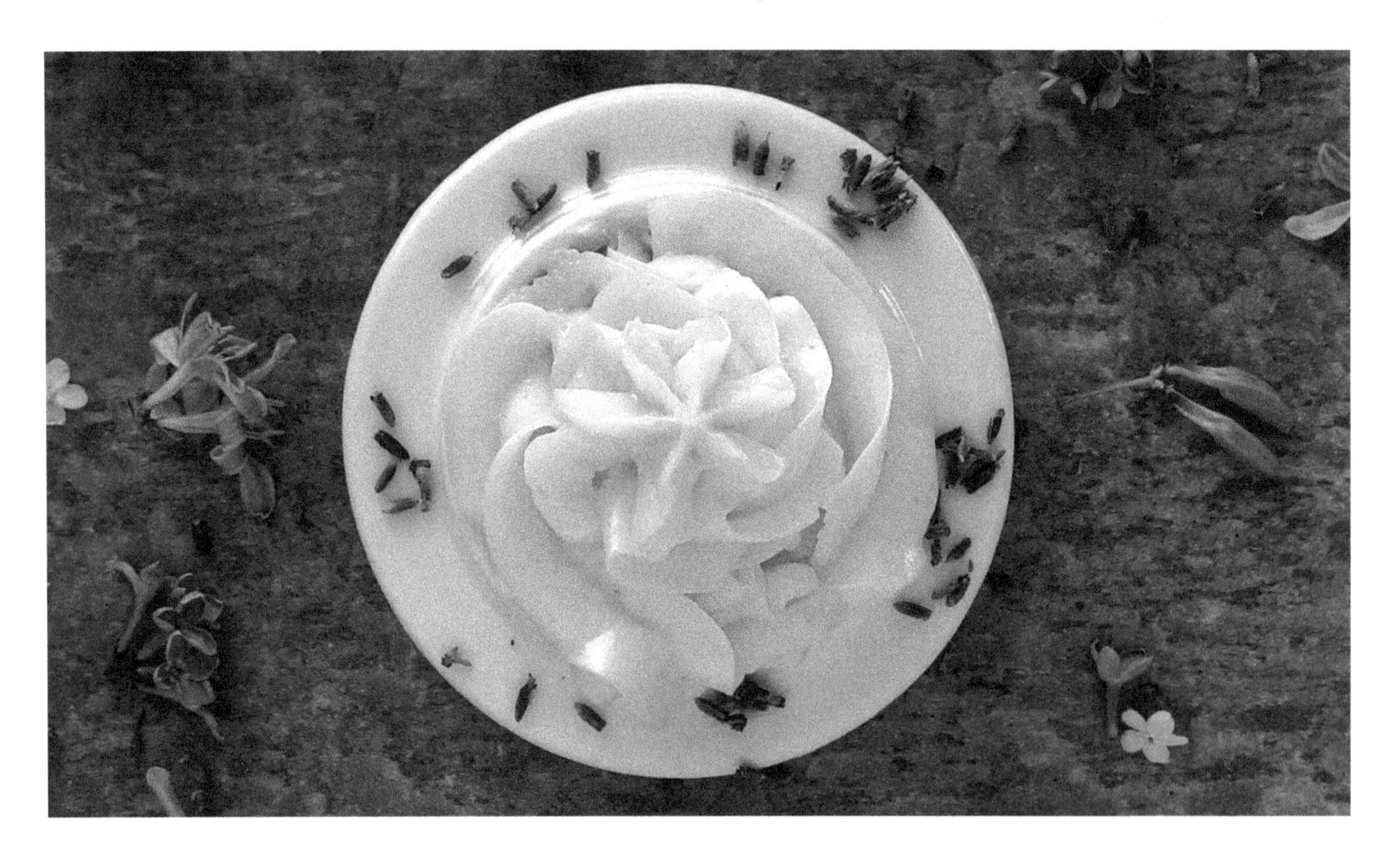

This light whipped moisturizer can be scented with any essential oil. Vanilla-lavender is calming to the senses and my personal favourite.

(Makes one small jar)

Equipment list

- Small 8-oz mason jar container with lid
- 1 glass measuring cup
- Food processor

Ingredients

- ¼ cup shea butter
- ¼ cup coconut oil (semi-hard)
- ¼ cup jojoba oil
- 8 drops lavender essential oil
- 6 drops vanilla essential oil

Instructions

You can melt the shea butter in a microwave or on the stove top.

For the microwave

1. Measure out the shea butter, and coconut oil and add to the glass measuring cup.
2. Microwave for 45 seconds, stir, and microwave again for 30 seconds.
3. Continue microwaving in 30-second intervals until the mixture is completely melted.
4. Once melted add the jojoba oil and essential oil and pour into clean dry, glass jars.
5. Let set for several hours or overnight. Store in a cool place.

For the stove top

1. Fill a medium-sized clean pot with 3 to 4 cups water. Place on the stove burner.
2. Measure out the shea butter, and coconut oil and add to the glass measuring cup.
3. Place your glass measuring cup in the pot of water.
4. Turn on the stove to medium-low setting. Turn the numbered dial to about four. This method heats slowly and does not scorch the ingredients.
5. With a metal spoon, stir constantly. Never leave the oils unattended.
6. Once your mixture is completely melted (about 15 minutes), turn off the stove and carefully remove the glass cup from the pot of water. Stir in jojoba oil and essential oil.
7. Fill your glass container, and let set for several hours or overnight. Store in a cool place.

Tip

You can add more essential oils for a stronger scent.
To give your body whip a light, fluffy whipping, you must scoop the chilled body whip into a clean, dry, food processor. Blend for 1-2 minutes.
Scoop back into the jar, or pipe with an icing bag.

Fresh Lemon-Coconut Body Whip

A little jar of sunshine

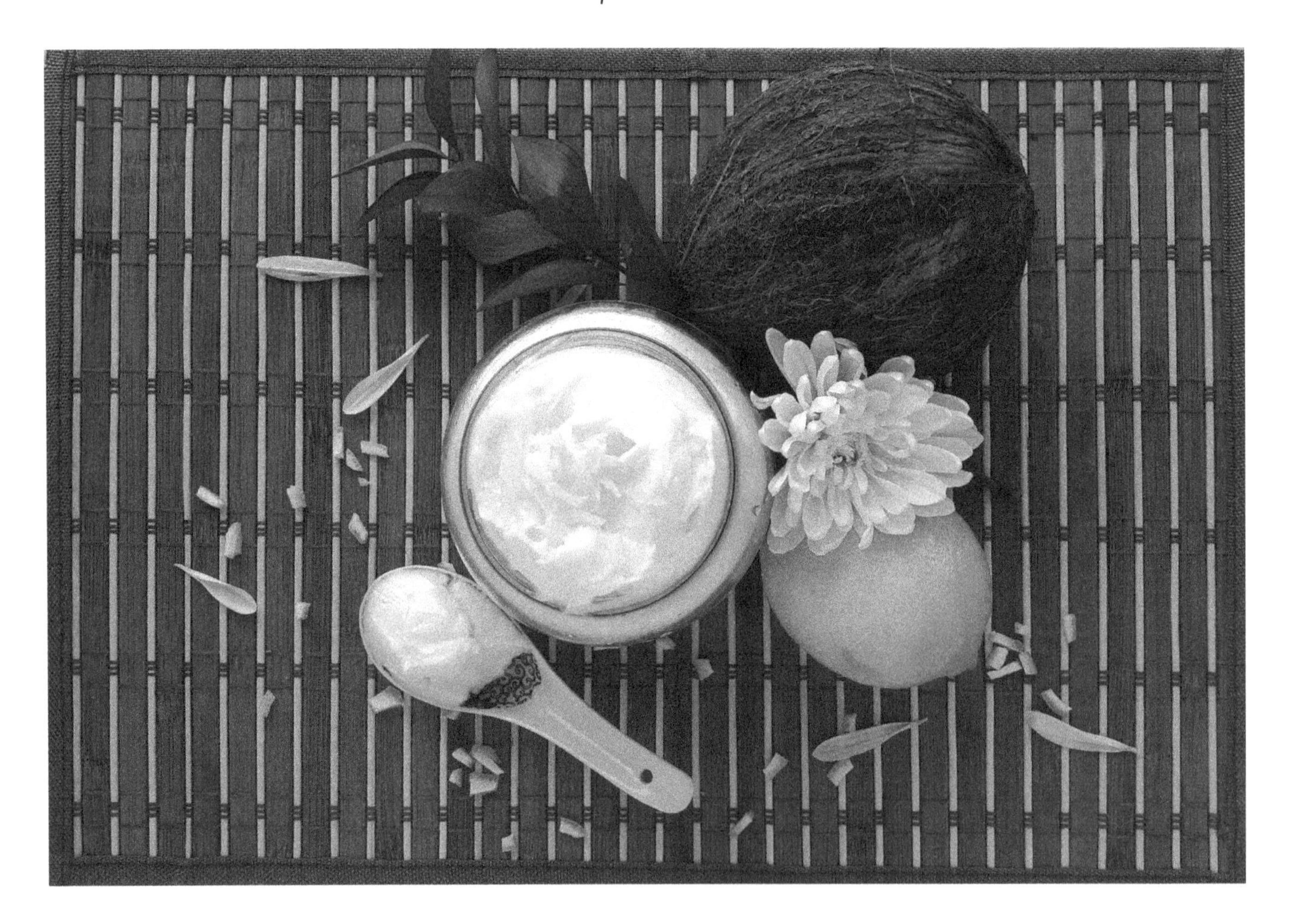

Need a little morning pick up? Lemon is a terrific mood and energy booster. This is a clean tropical scent.

(Makes one small jar)

Equipment list

- Small 8-oz mason jar with lid
- 1 glass measuring cup
- Food processor

Ingredients

- ¼ cup shea butter
- ¼ cup coconut oil (semi-hard)
- ¼ cup jojoba oil
- 1 tsp pure coconut extract
- 12 drops lemon essential oil

Instructions

You can melt the shea butter in a microwave or on the stove top.

For the microwave

1. Measure out the shea butter, and coconut oil and add to the glass measuring cup.
2. Microwave for 45 seconds, stir, and microwave again for 30 seconds.
3. Continue microwaving in 30-second intervals until the mixture is completely melted.
4. Stir in jojoba oil, coconut extract, essential oils, and then pour into clean, dry glass jars.
5. Let set for several hours or overnight. Store in a cool place.

For the stove top

1. Fill a medium-sized clean pot with 3 to 4 cups water. Place on the stove burner.
2. Measure out the shea butter, and coconut oil and add to the glass measuring cup.
3. Place your glass measuring cup in the pot of water.
4. Turn on the stove to medium-low setting. Turn the numbered dial to about four. This method heats slowly and does not scorch the ingredients.

5. With a metal spoon, stir constantly. Never leave the oils unattended.
6. Once your mixture is completely melted (about 15 minutes), turn off the stove and carefully remove the glass cup from the pot of water.
7. Stir in the jojoba oil, coconut extract, and essential oil. Fill your glass container, and let set for several hours or overnight. Store in a cool place.

Tip

You can add more essential oils for a stronger scent.
To give your body whip a light, fluffy whipping, you must scoop the chilled body whip into a clean, dry, food processor. Blend for 1-2 minutes.
Scoop back into the jar, or pipe with an icing bag

BODY SPRAY
Smell Amazing Without Chemicals

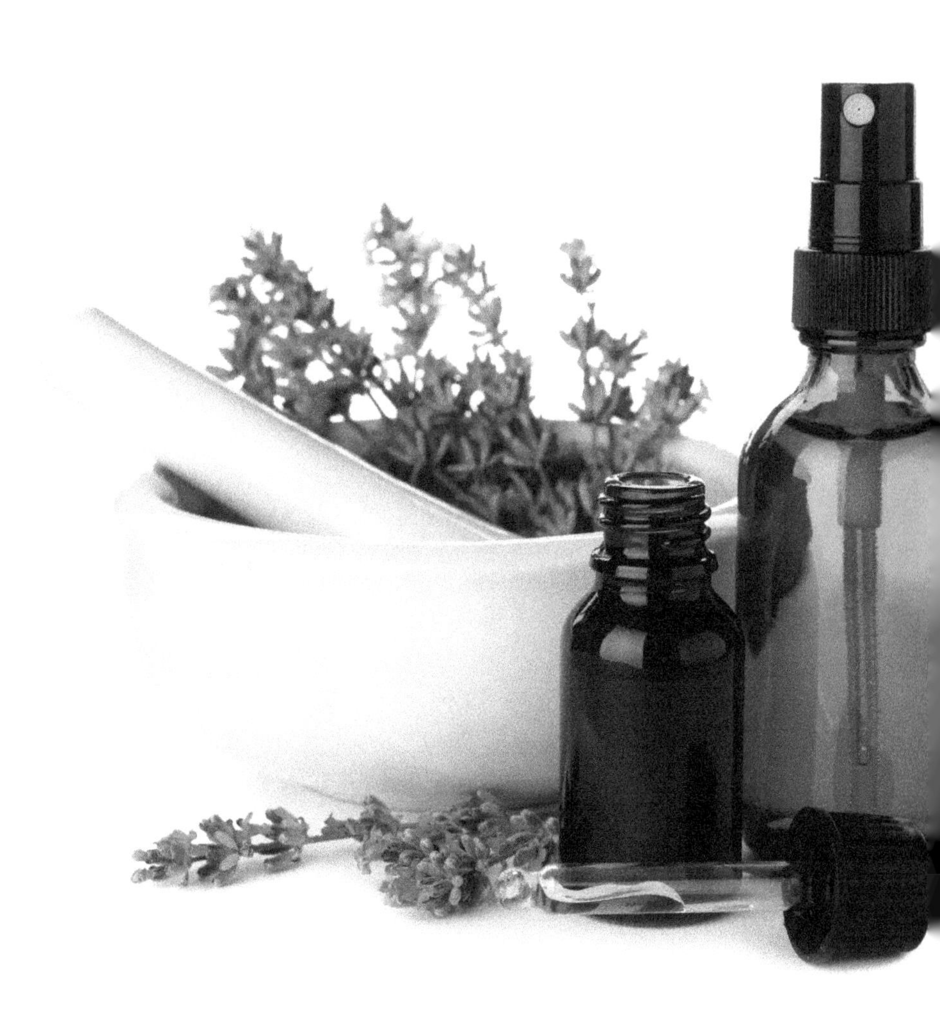

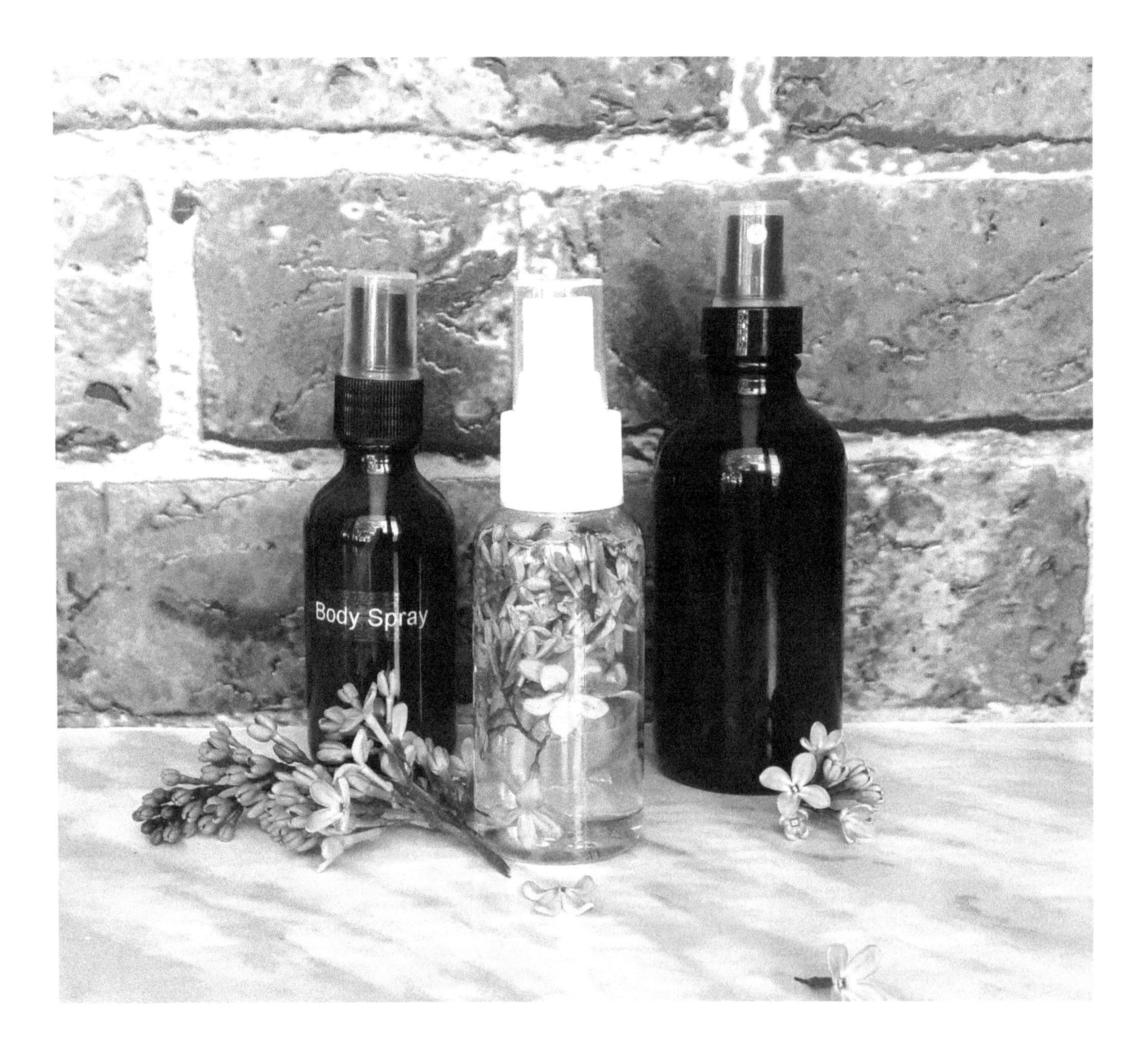
Body Spray

Body spray is much like perfume but made to be sprayed all over the body. Usually body sprays are inexpensive because they contain cheap, synthetic fragrances that can cause allergic reactions and headaches. The hazard is they require a propellant chemical to turn the liquid into an aerosol spray. As mentioned in an earlier chapter, aerosols are harmful to us and our environment. The chemicals used in these popular body sprays have dire consequences.

Commercial body sprays contain a slurry of harmful chemicals that are linked to cancer, hormonal problems, and infertility. This is *not* a product you want to be using. I will show you how to make an amazing manly body spray that mimics these products but without the chemicals.

Enjoy my easy DIY body sprays that smell fresh and clean, and contain only natural ingredients.

Men's Natural Body Spray

A healthier alternative to AXE body spray

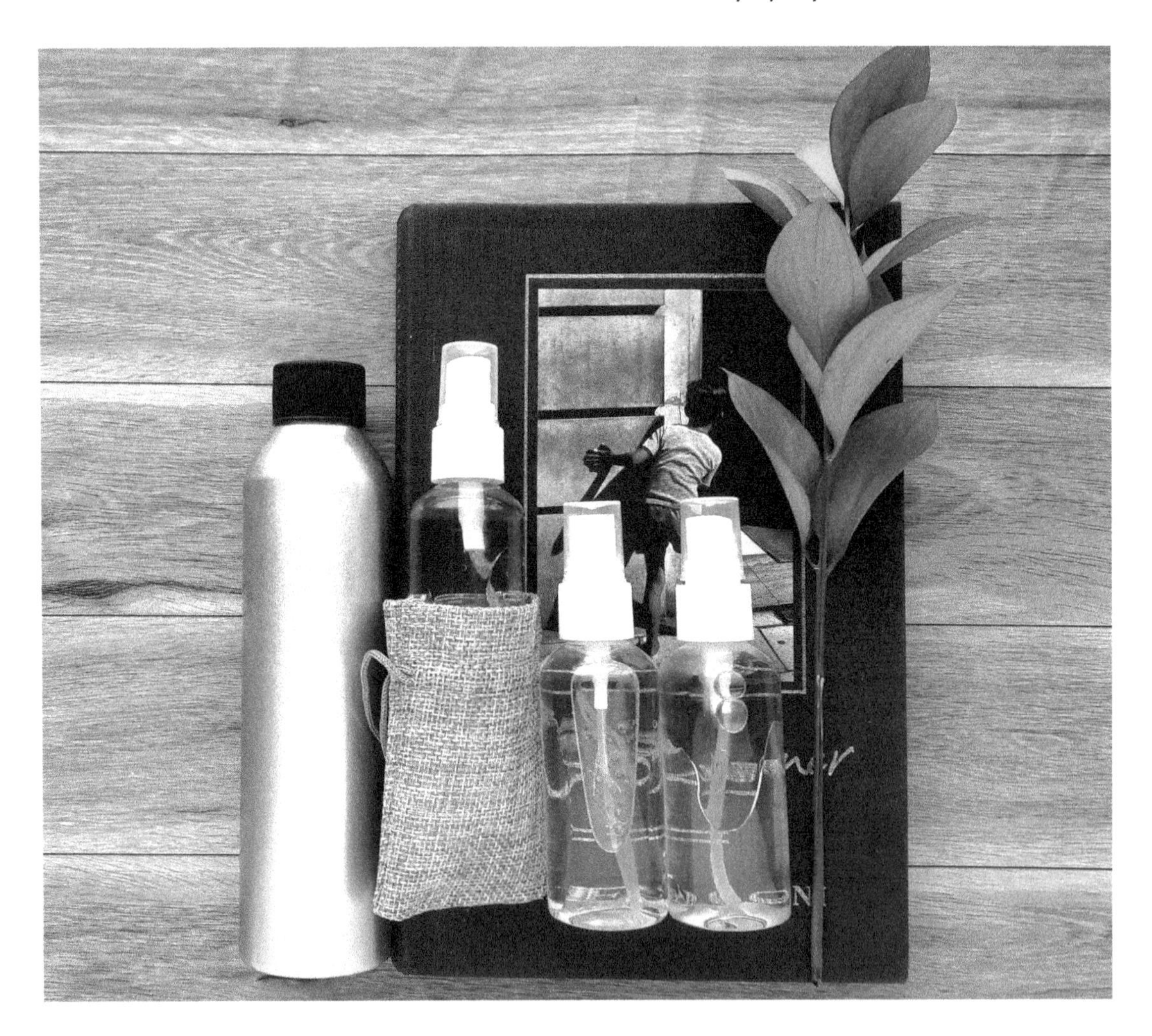

(Makes one 4 oz spray bottle)

Equipment list

- Clean, empty 4-oz spray bottle
- Small funnel

Ingredients

- 2 TBSP vodka or any type of grain alcohol
- 1 tsp vegetable glycerin
- Filtered water
- Essential oils: 20 drops orange, 10 drops vanilla, 10 drops cedarwood, 4 drops lemon, 4 drops ylang ylang

Instructions

1. In a clean glass measuring cup, mix everything except the water.
2. Carefully pour through a funnel into the clean spray bottle.
3. Fill the rest of the bottle with water.

Tip

The vodka naturally preserves the body spray and helps distribute the spray. This will last many months.

Men's Fresh and Clean Body Spray

Citrus and woodsy

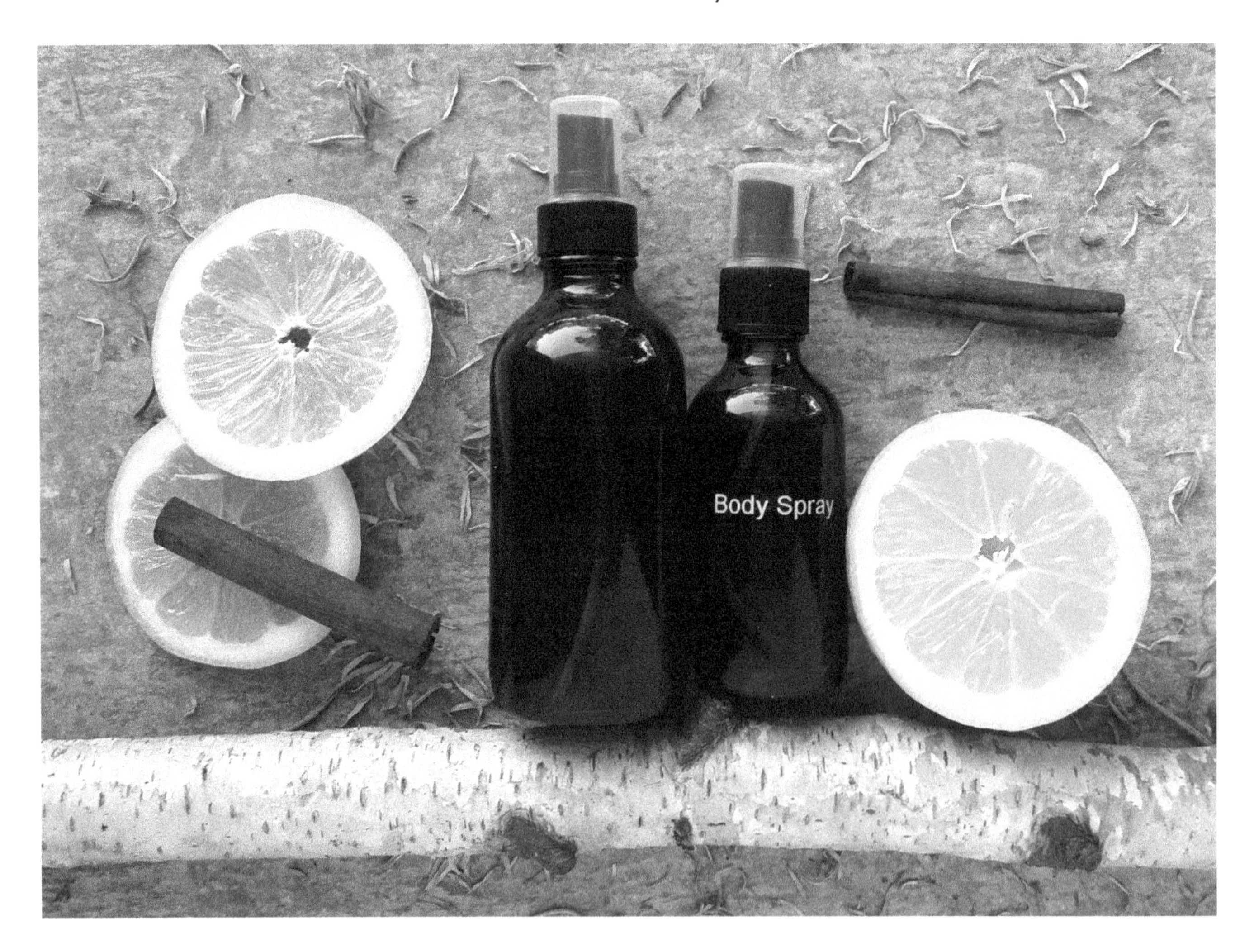

(Makes one 4 oz spray bottle)

Equipment list

- Clean, empty 4-oz spray bottle
- Small funnel

Ingredients

- 2 TBSP vodka or any type of grain alcohol
- 1 tsp vegetable glycerin
- Filtered water
- Essential oils: 20 drops orange, 12 drops lemon, 8 drops grapefruit, 8 drops cedarwood

Instructions

1. In a clean glass measuring cup, mix everything except the water.
2. Carefully pour through a funnel into the clean spray bottle.
3. Fill the rest of the bottle with water.

Tip

The vodka naturally preserves the body spray and helps distribute the spray. This will last many months.

Women's Floral Body Spray

Fresh and revitalizing

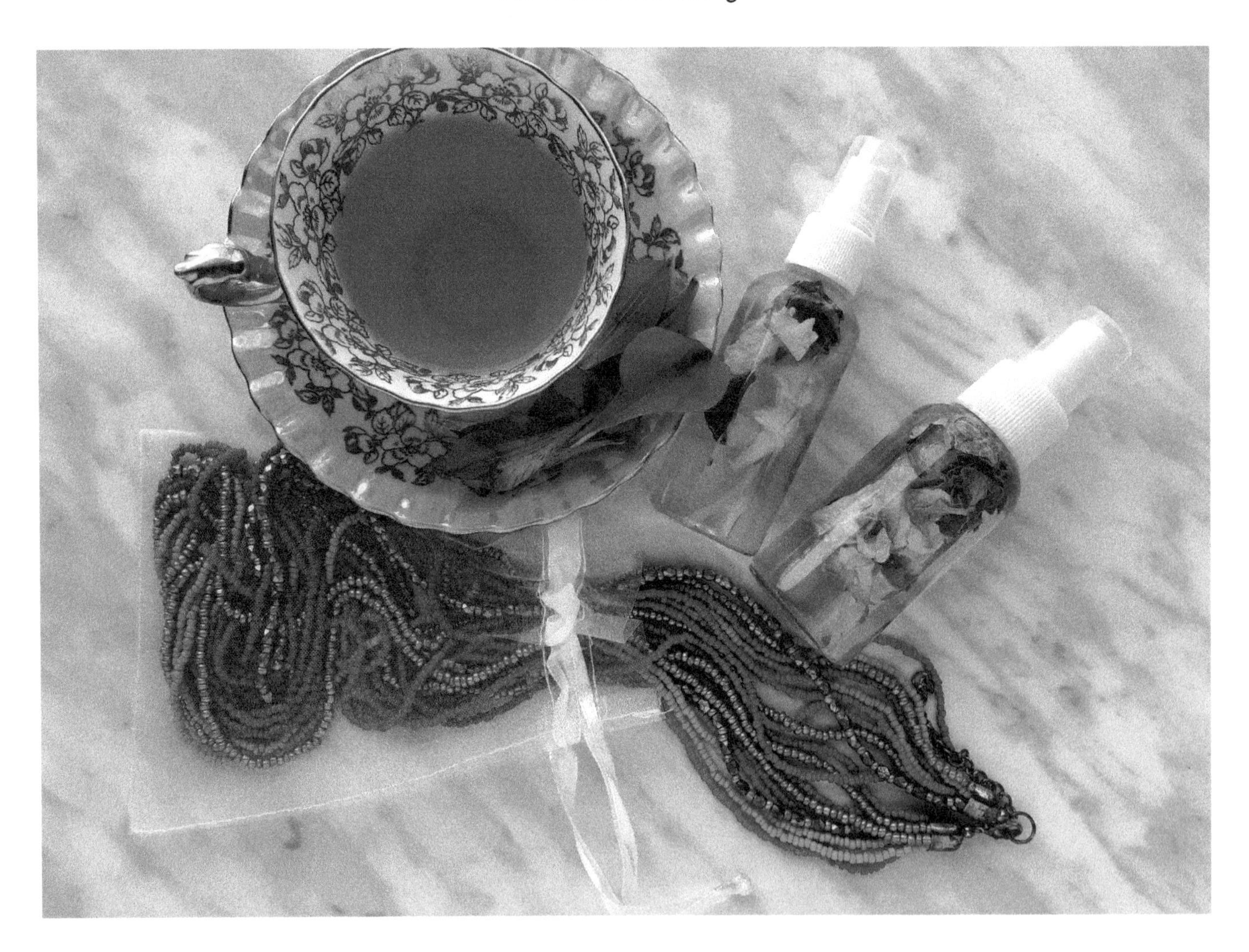

(Makes one 4 oz spray bottle)

Equipment list

- Clean, empty 4-oz spray bottle
- Small funnel

Ingredients

- 2 TBSP vodka or any type of grain alcohol
- 1 tsp vegetable glycerin
- Filtered water
- Essential oils: 15 drops rose, 15 drops lilac or lily, 10 drops orange, 8 drops lemon

Instructions

1. In a clean glass measuring cup, mix all ingredients, except the water.
2. Carefully pour through a funnel into the clean spray bottle.
3. Fill the rest of the bottle with water.

Tip

The vodka naturally preserves the body spray and helps distribute the spray. This will last many months.

Women's Sensual Body Spray

Warm and spicy

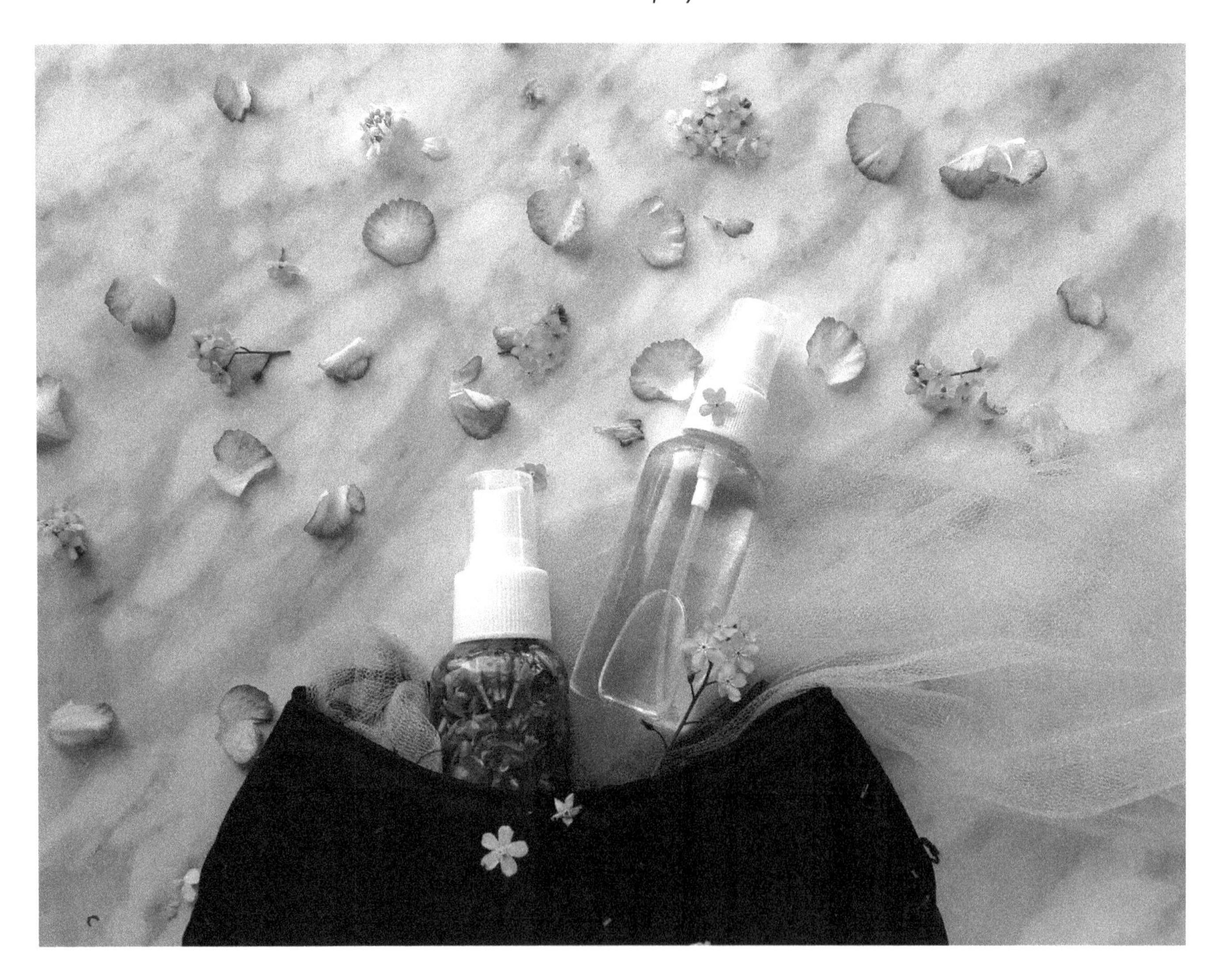

(Makes one 4 oz spray bottle)

Equipment list

- Clean, empty 4-oz spray bottle
- Small funnel

Ingredients

- 2 TBSP vodka or any type of grain alcohol
- 1 tsp vegetable glycerin
- Filtered water
- Essential oils: 25 drops vanilla, 10 drops cinnamon, 10 drops orange, 3 drops neroli

Instructions

1. In a clean glass measuring cup, mix all ingredients.
2. Carefully pour through a funnel into the spray bottle.
3. Fill the rest of the bottle with water.

Tip

The vodka naturally preserves the body spray and helps distribute the spray. This will last many months.

BATH AND SHOWER TIME
Get Clean Naturally

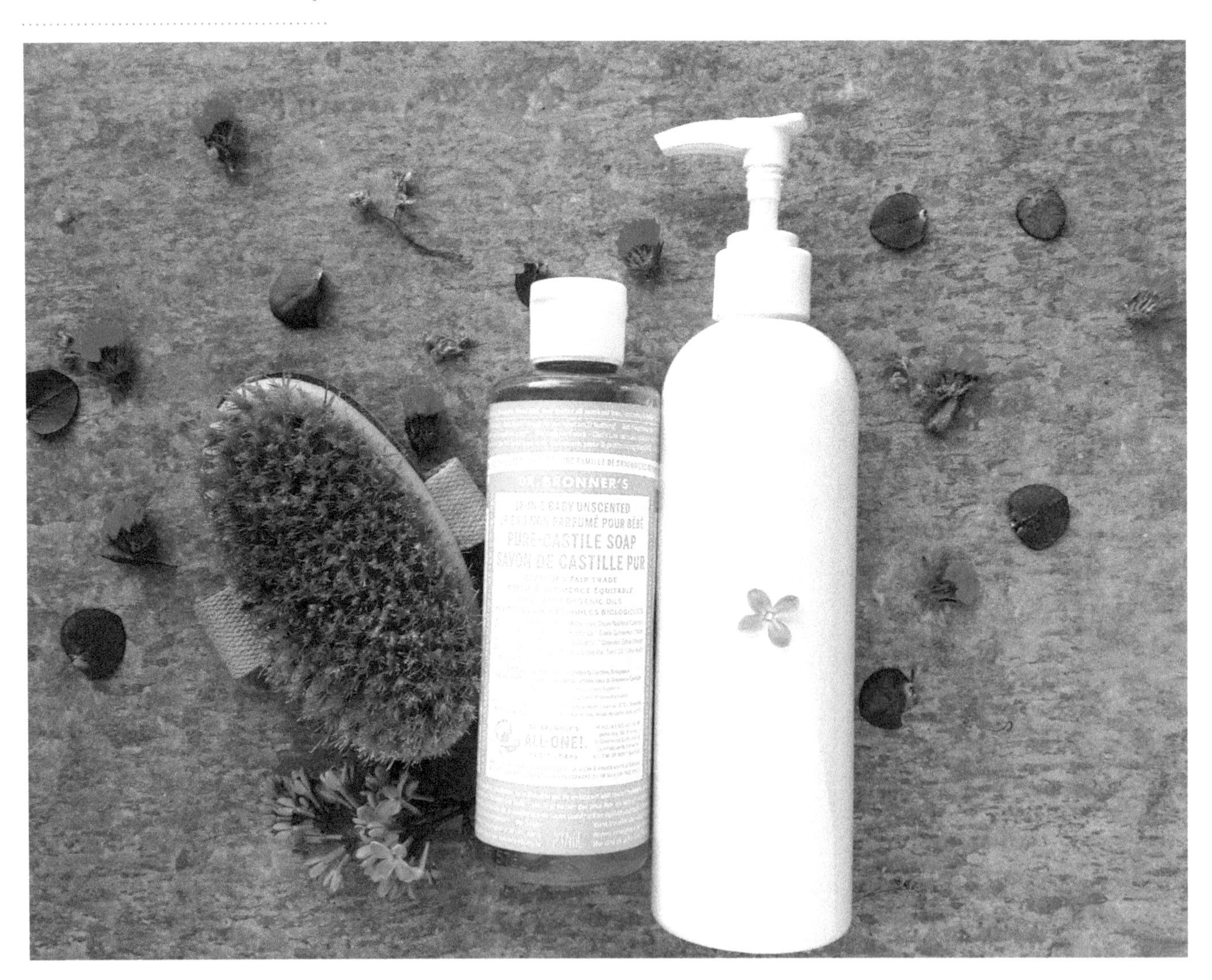

Whether you bathe or shower, it's important to use natural products. Here's why. When we immerse ourselves in hot water, our pores open wide and quickly absorb whatever we apply to ourselves. Shampoos and body wash contain many chemicals, such as parabens and sulfites. Bubble bath, bath oils, and commercially made bath bombs have a long-lasting scent only found through the use of synthetic fragrance. Sadly, even baby products touted as gentler contain many harmful components. We definitely don't want that for our kids.

The good news is you can still enjoy bath and shower time while using all-natural ingredients. I like to infuse bath products with essential oils. This way we can enjoy the healing benefits of aromatherapy.

Basically, any of the bath products found in stores contains ingredients on the naughty list. Commonly found ingredients are sodium laureth sulfate, disodium laureth sulfosuccinate, artificial colours, and fragrance.

Enjoy these recipes for shower gel, bath salts, and bath fizz. They are so much fun to make and you can really get creative here.

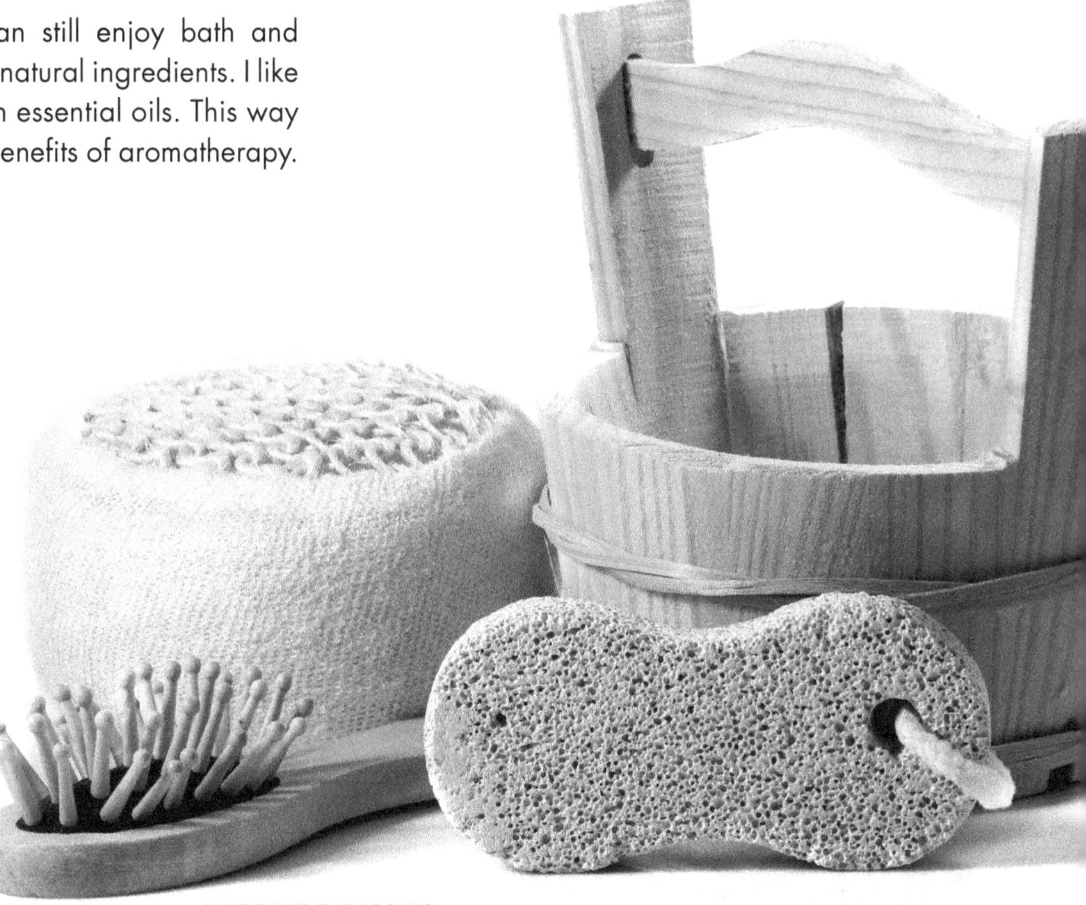

Easy Bath and Shower Gel

Gentle for all skin types

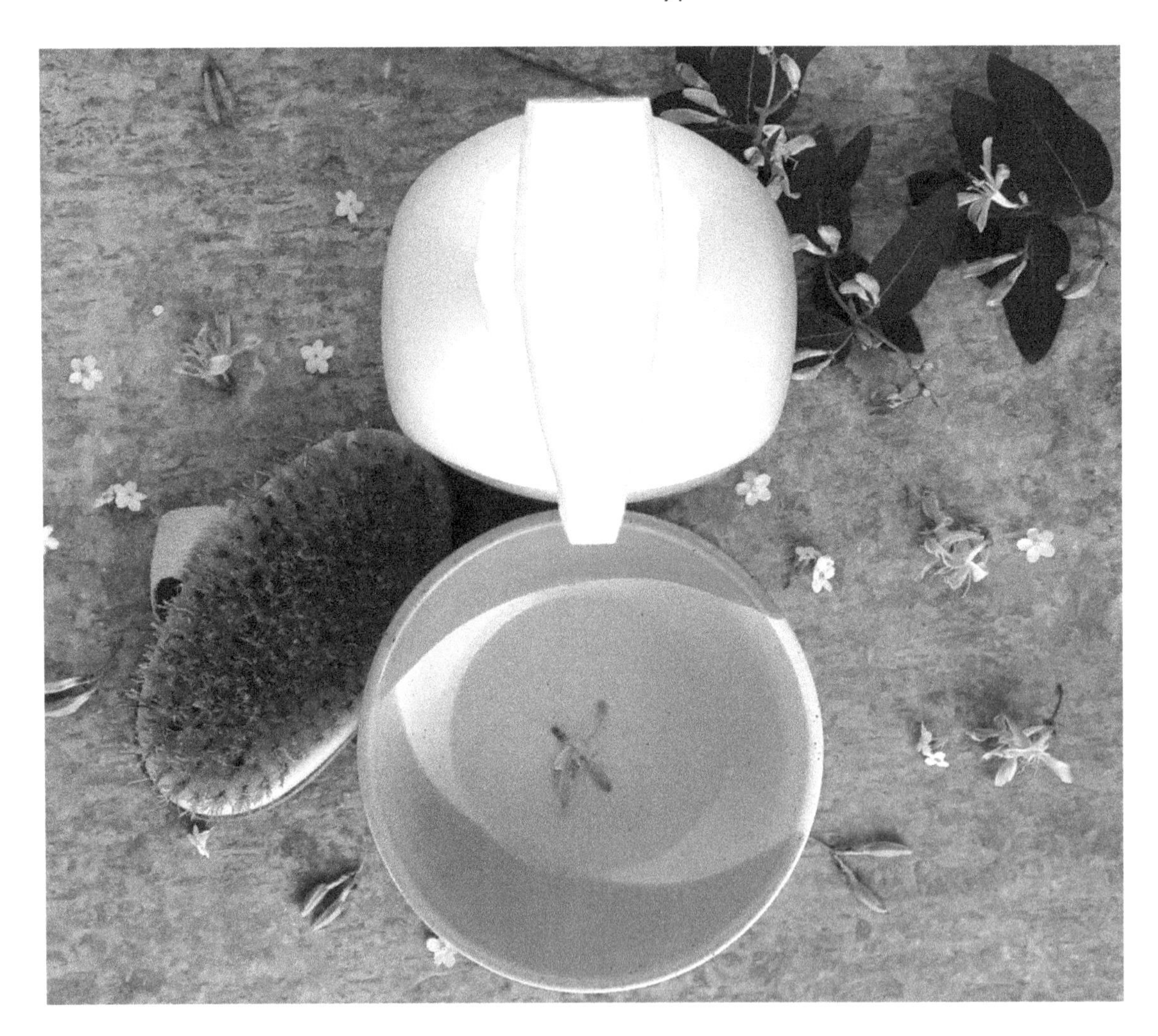

(Makes one 12 oz container)

Equipment list

- 12-oz container with pump or dispenser

Ingredients

- 1 cup liquid castile soap (unscented)
- 1 TBSP vegetable glycerin
- 2 TBSP water
- 2 TBSP jojoba oil
- 1 tsp vitamin E oil
- 1 tsp essential oil(s) of your choice

Instructions

1. Mix all of the ingredients together and store in a pump bottle.
2. Shake gently.

Morning Wake-Up Shower Gel

Invigorating

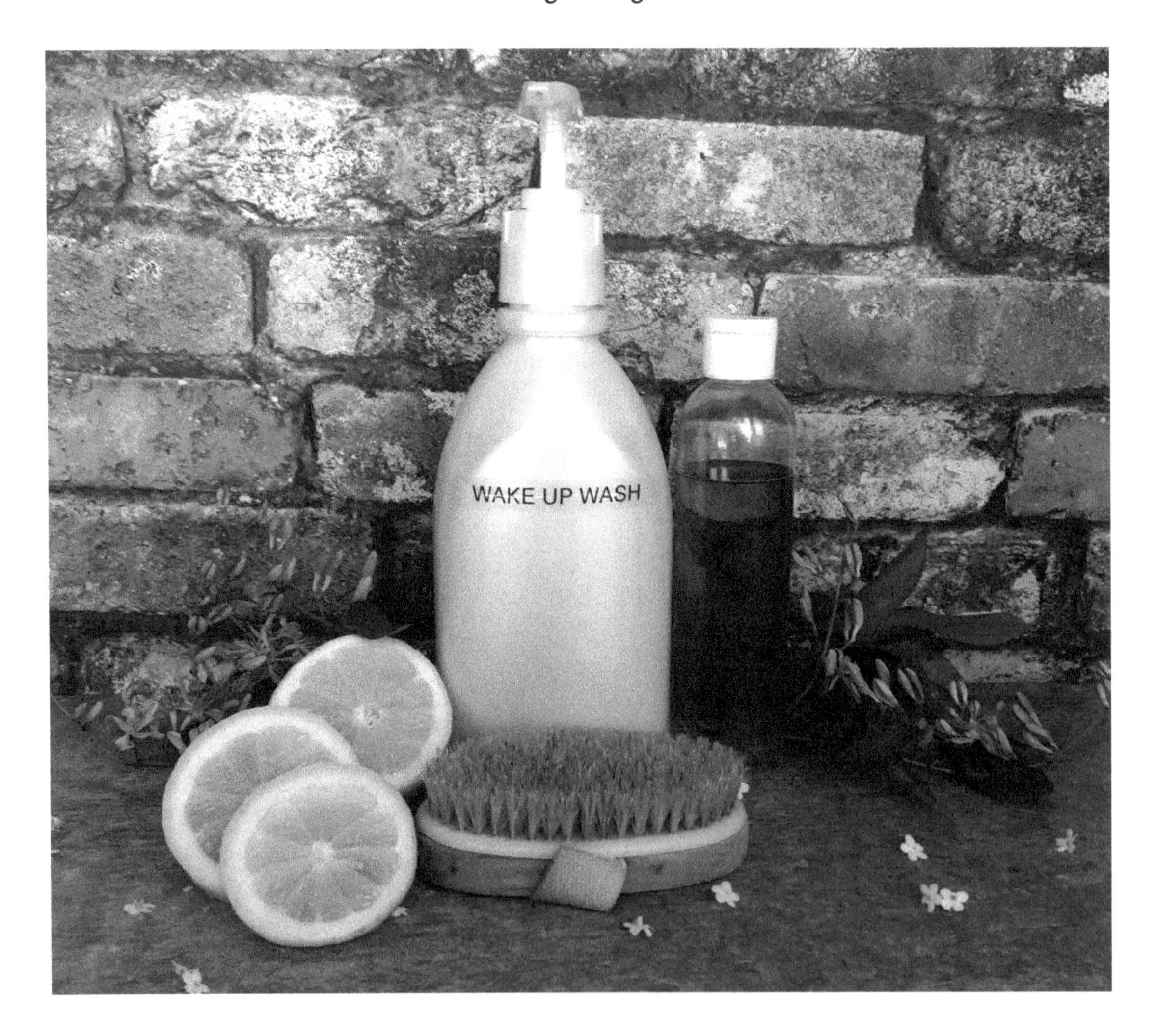

(Makes one 12 oz container)

Equipment list

- 12-oz container with pump or dispenser

Ingredients

- 1 cup liquid castile soap (unscented)
- 1 TBSP vegetable glycerin
- 2 TBSP water
- 2 tsp jojoba oil
- 1 tsp vitamin E oil
- Essential oils: 40 drops orange, 30 drops lemon, 15 drops peppermint

Instructions

1. Mix all of the ingredients together and store in a pump bottle.
2. Shake gently.

Luxurious Bath Oil

Cleopatra would love this!

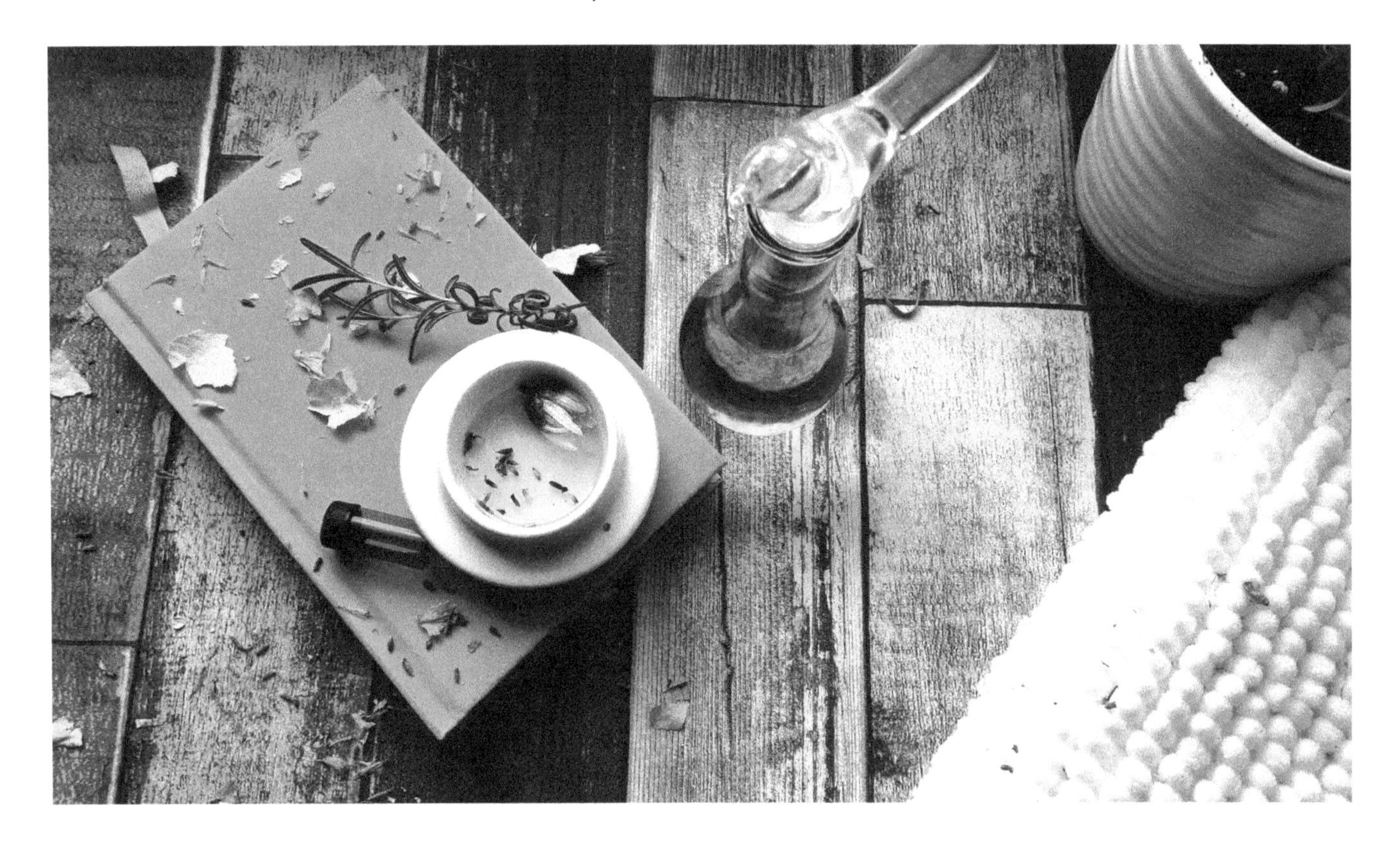

Enjoy this aromatherapy bath, complete with fragrant oils to quiet your mind. Your body will feel smooth and silky all day!

(Makes one 8 oz jar)

Equipment list

- 8-oz mason jar or glass container with lid

Ingredients

- ½ cup olive oil
- ½ cup sweet almond oil
- 1 tsp essential oil(s) of your choice

Option additions

- Crushed flower petals
- Lavender flowers
- Dried teas

Instructions

1. Mix the olive and almond oils together.
2. Add the desired essential oils. (See our recommendations below.)
   Stir in any optional dried flowers or tea, or omit.

Cheer up: basil, bergamot, jasmine, rose
Detoxing: sandalwood, rosemary, sage
Energizing: lemon, orange, bergamot
Relaxing: lavender, chamomile oil
Sensual: rose, neroli, ylang ylang

Tip

Add ¼ cup of the bath oil to your bath water. Soak for 20 minutes or as desired.

DIY Relaxing Bath Salts

Detox your body

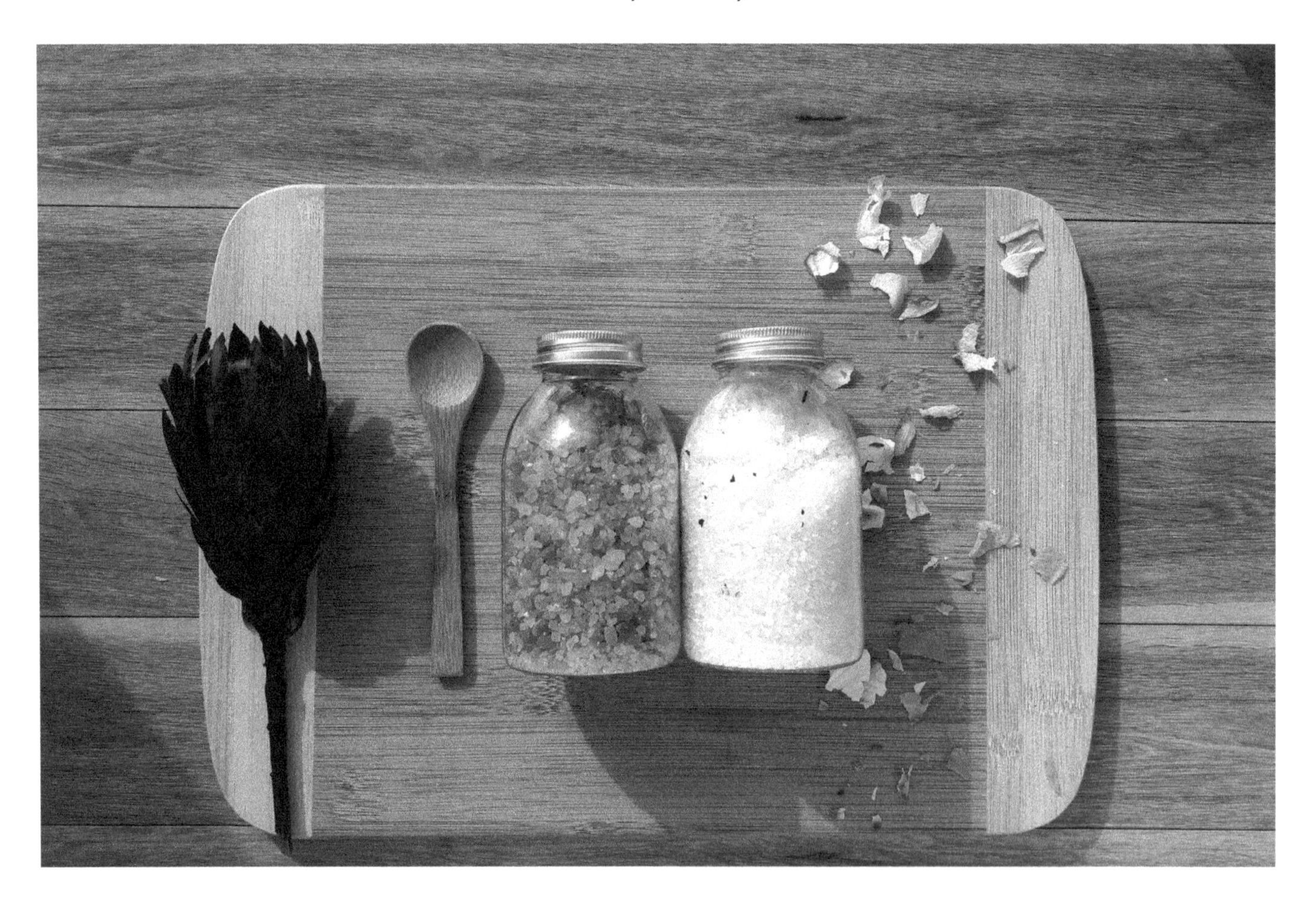

Epsom salts are a great way to detox your body, reduce cellulite and puffiness, and help you relax after a long day.

(Makes one 8 oz jar)

Equipment list

- 8-oz mason jar or glass container with lid

Ingredients

- 1 cup Epsom salts
- 1 TBSP carrier oil (jojoba, grapeseed, or sweet almond)
- 1 tsp of your favourite essential oil

Optional additions

- Dried flowers
- Dried tea leaves
- Dried mint
- Natural colour

Instructions

1. In a glass bowl, add the Epsom salts.
2. Measure out the carrier oil and add to the salts.
3. Add 1 tsp of your preferred essential oil and any optional additions.
4. Mix well and store in glass jar with lid.

Tips

If you'd like to make your salts look "pretty," you can add dried flowers, mint, tea leaves, etc., but bear in mind they will float in the bath water and be on your skin. It can be a bit messy but certainly looks lovely if giving as a gift.

Add ½ cup of the bath salts to your bath water. Soak for 20 minutes or more.

Fun fact

Epsom salts were discovered in Epsom, England, in the 1800s. These salts contain magnesium, which relaxes the muscles.

Lavender Bath Salts

Surrender to relaxation

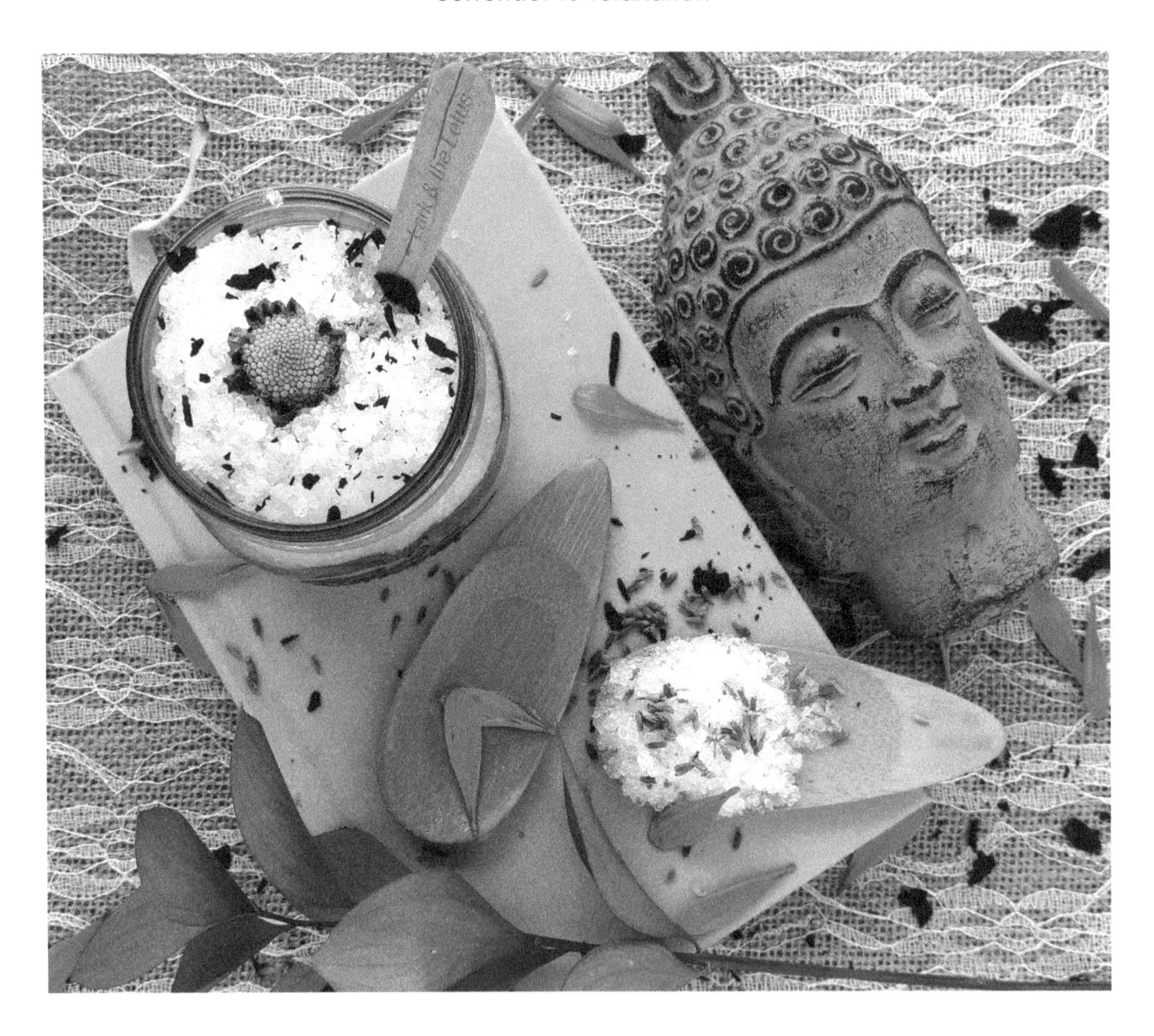

(Makes one 8 oz jar)

Equipment list

- 8-oz mason jar or glass container with lid

Ingredients

- 1 cup Epsom salts
- 1 TBSP carrier oil (jojoba)
- 1 tsp lavender essential oil
- ¼ cup dried lavender flowers

Instructions

1. In a glass bowl, add the Epsom salts.
2. Add the jojoba oil, essential oil, and flowers.
3. Mix well and store in glass jar with lid.

Tips

Best used within 30 days.

Add ½ cup of the bath salts to your bath water. Soak for 20 minutes or more.

Fresh Grapefruit Bath Salts

Uplifting

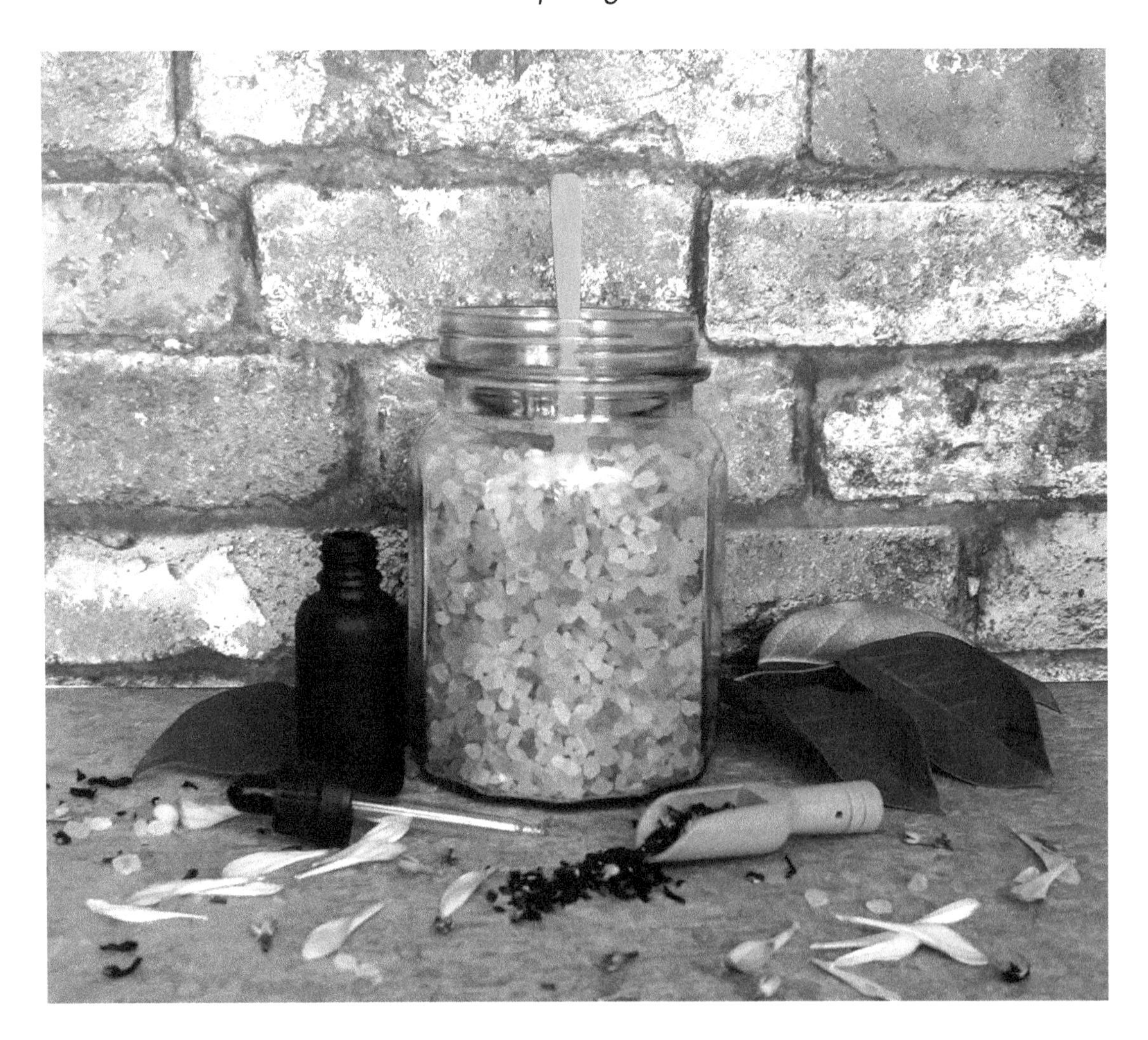

(Makes one 8 oz jar)

Equipment list

- 8-oz mason jar or glass container with lid

Ingredients

- ½ cup Epsom salts
- ½ cup pink Himalayan salts (medium fine)
- 1 TBSP carrier oil (sweet almond)
- 1 tsp grapefruit essential oil
- ¼ cup dried hibiscus tea

Instructions

1. In a glass bowl, add the Epsom and Himalayan salts.
2. Add the almond oil, essential oil, and dried tea.
3. Mix well and store in glass jar with lid.

Tips

Best used within 30 days.

Add ½ cup of the bath salts to your bath water. Soak for 20 minutes or more.

Fizzy Bath Powder

Designed your way

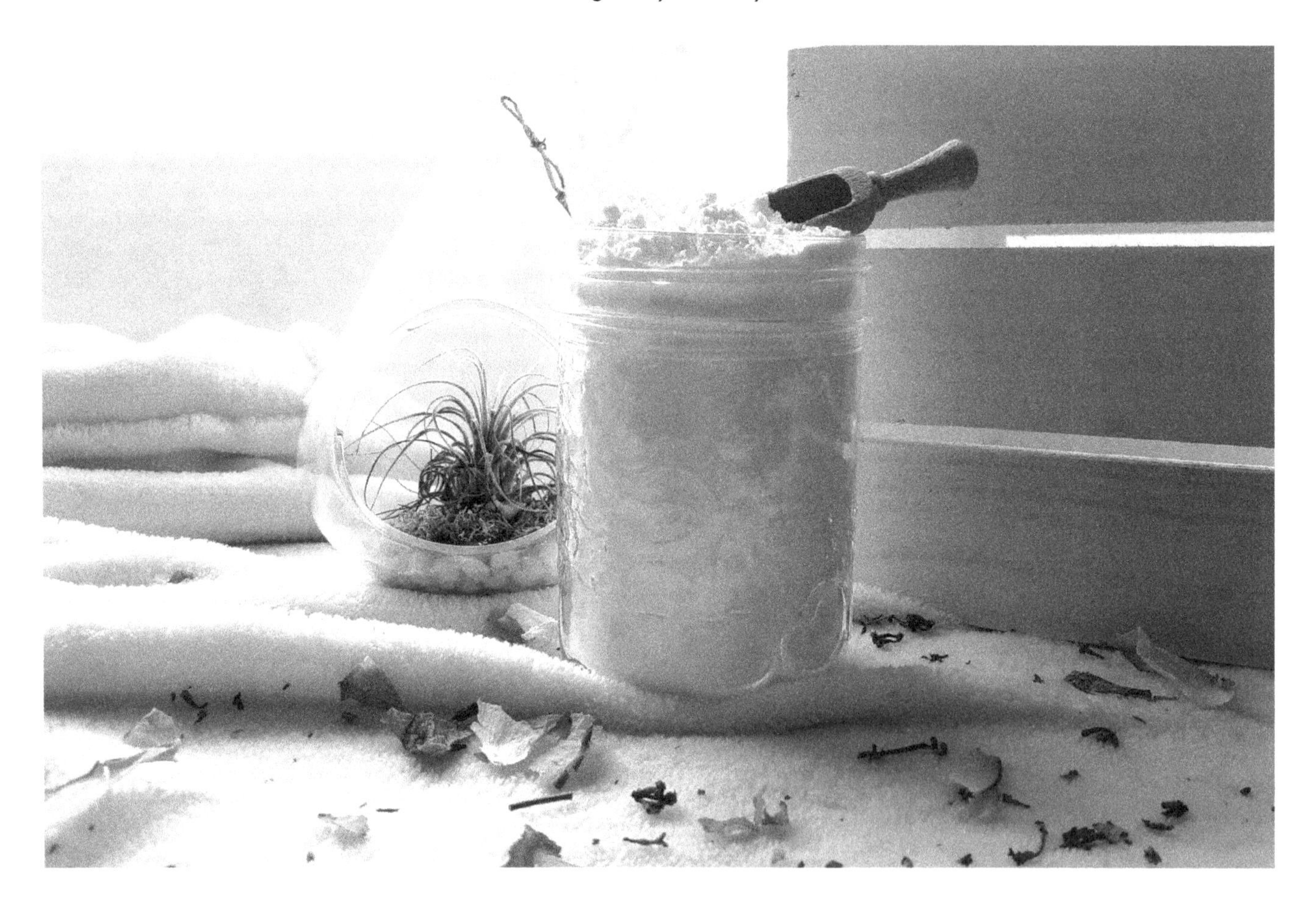

This has the same effect as a bath bomb but will yield several baths if you store it in a mason jar. Colour and scent are customizable, so have fun with it!

(Makes two 8 oz jars)

Equipment list

- Two 8-oz mason jars or glass containers with lids
- Small scoop

Ingredients

- 1 cup baking soda
- ½ cup cornstarch or skim milk powder
- ½ cup citric acid
- 1 tsp essential oil of your choice

Optional additions

- 1 tsp natural colour extract (beetroot, hibiscus, matcha, etc.)
- 1 tsp dried flowers, mint, tea leaves

Instructions

1. In a glass bowl, add the soda, starch, and citric acid.
2. Add the essential oil and any optional additions. Stir well to get out any lumps.
3. Add any optional dried flowers or extracts, or omit.
4. Scoop into glass jars with lids.

Tips

Best used within 30 days.

Add ½ cup of the bath fizz to your bath water. Watch the water fizz! Soak for 20 minutes or more.

Cupcake Bath Fizz

Smells just like cake!

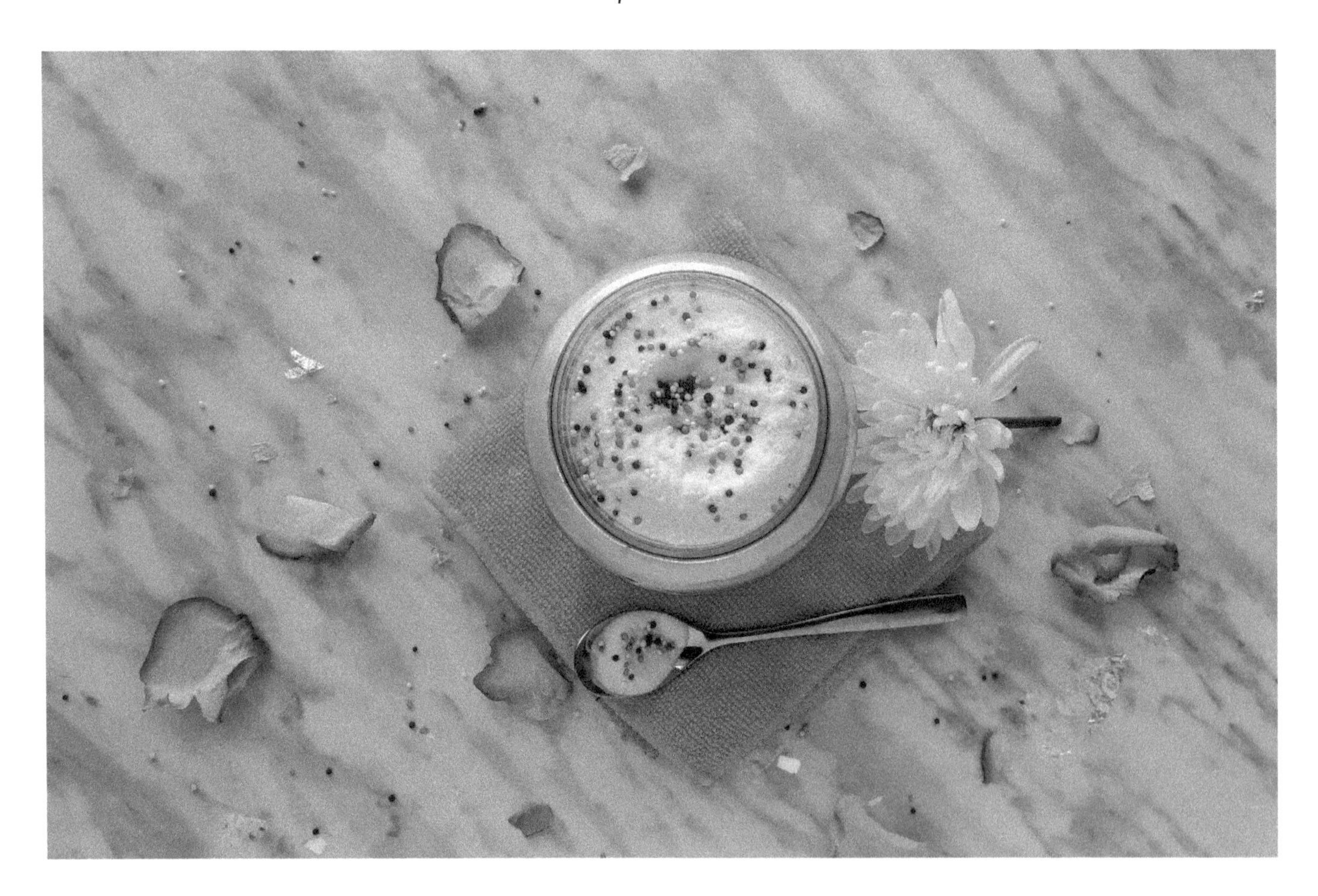

(Makes one 8 oz jar)

Equipment list

- 8-oz mason jar or glass container with lid
- Small scoop

Ingredients

- 1 cup baking soda
- ½ cup corn starch
- ½ cup citric acid
- Essential oils: 50 drops vanilla, 20 drops cinnamon, 10 drops lemon, 3 drops orange
- 1 tsp hibiscus powder or beetroot powder
- 2 TBSP cake sprinkles

Instructions

1. In a glass bowl add the soda, starch, and citric acid.
2. Add the essential oils. Stir well to get out any lumps.
3. Next stir in hibiscus powder and cake sprinkles.
4. Scoop into glass jars with lids.

Tips

Best used within 30 days.

Add ½ cup of the bath fizz to your bath water.
Watch the water change colour as it fizzes. Soak for 20 minutes or more.

Cold and Flu Fighting Bath Fizz

Ease your congestion and aches

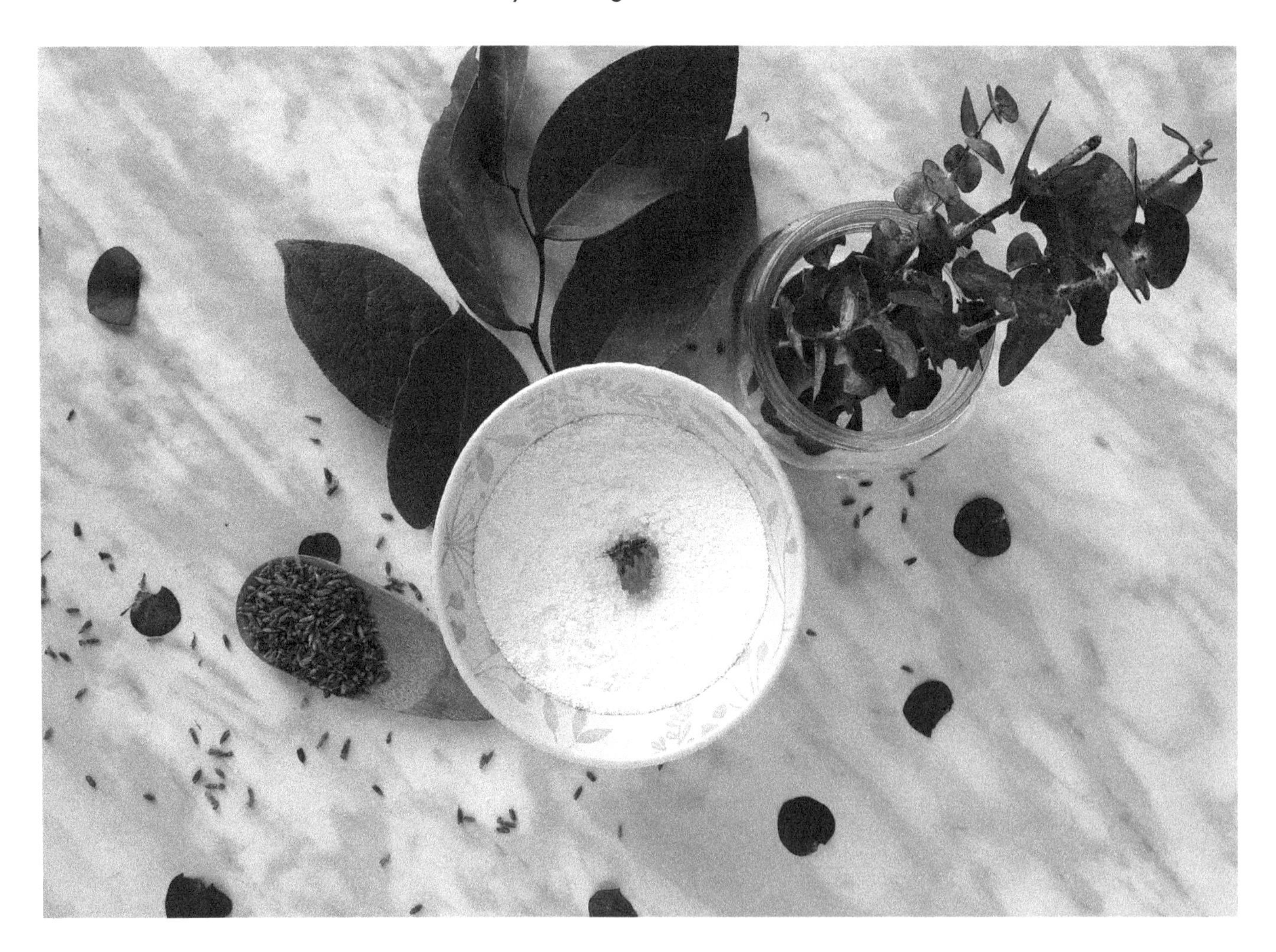

(Makes one 8 oz jar)

Equipment list

- 8-oz mason jar or glass container with lid
- Small scoop

Ingredients

- 1 cup baking soda
- ½ cup cornstarch
- ½ cup citric acid
- 2 TBSP Epsom salts
- Essential oils: 40 drops eucalyptus, 30 drops thyme, 10 drops peppermint, 5 drops lemon

Instructions

1. In a glass bowl, add the soda, starch, citric acid, and Epsom salts.
2. Add the essential oils. Stir well to get out any lumps.
3. Scoop into glass jar with lid.

Tips

Best used within 30 days.

Add ½ cup of the bath fizz to your bath water. Breathe deep and let the aromatherapy work its magic. Soak for 20 minutes or more.

SAFE FOR BABY AND KIDS

Items You Can Trust

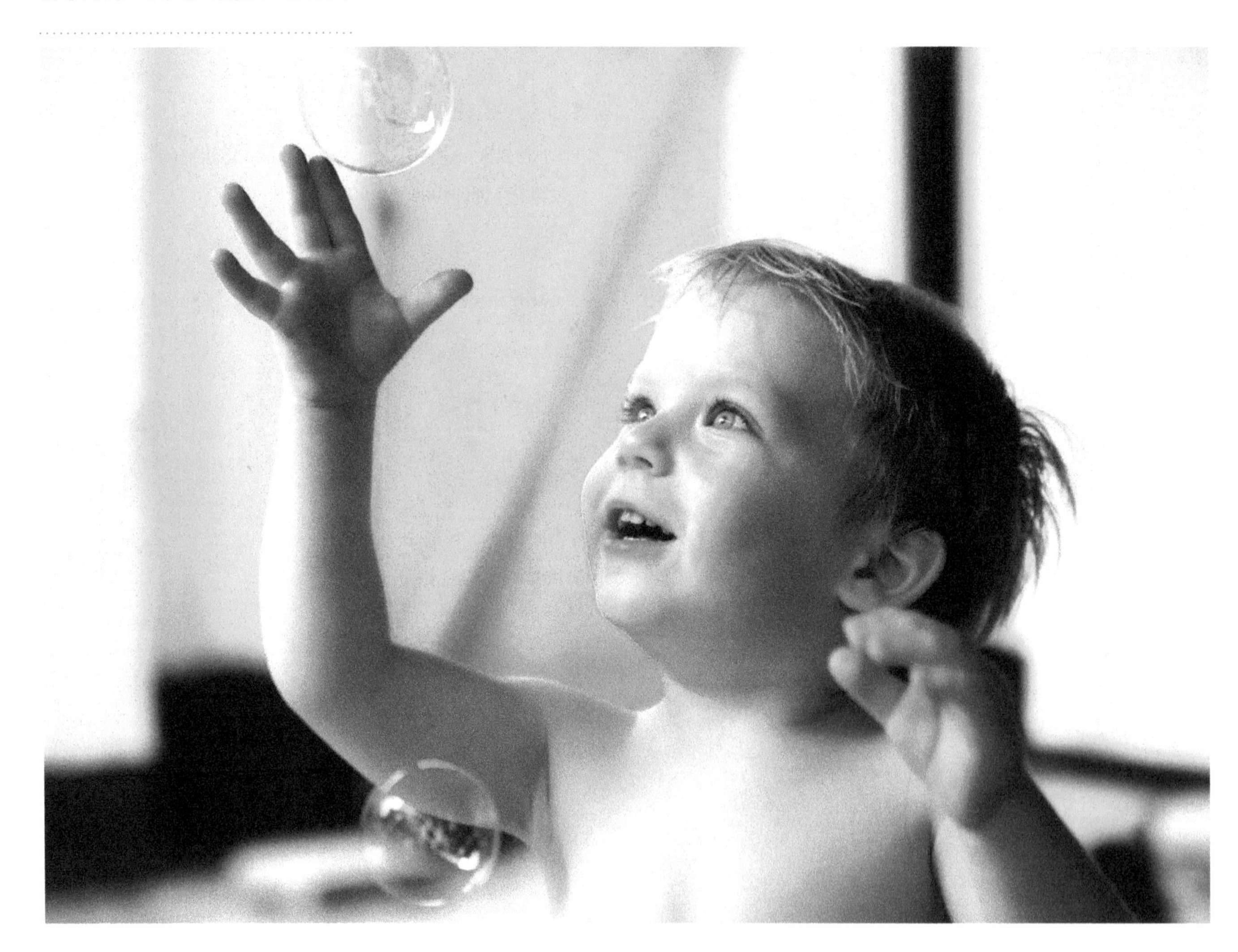

The baby industry is another booming area for personal care. We trust that these items are especially safe for baby, right? It's true that baby and kid products are made gentler and contain the least amounts of dyes, fragrance, and chemicals; however, they still contain many toxic preservatives and fragrant ingredients.

I urge you to take a closer look at the ingredients listed and make an informed decision before you purchase. Opt for fragrance-free, whenever and wherever possible. I will teach you how to make all of your favourite baby and kid products with organic and natural ingredients and NO chemicals!

I have included my best and gentlest baby recipes. I have not added any essential oils for scent to keep it as simple as possible. If you'd prefer to add a bit of scent, you can use baby-safe essentials oils such as lavender and chamomile.

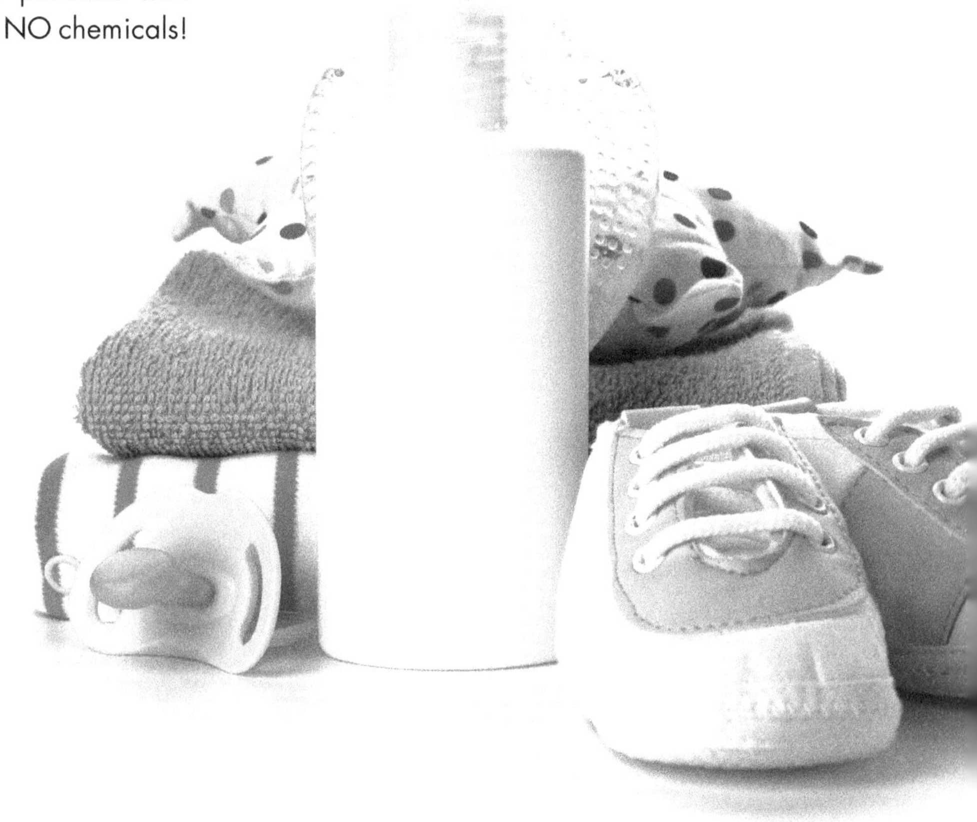

Gentle Talc-Free Baby Powder

Fresh and clean

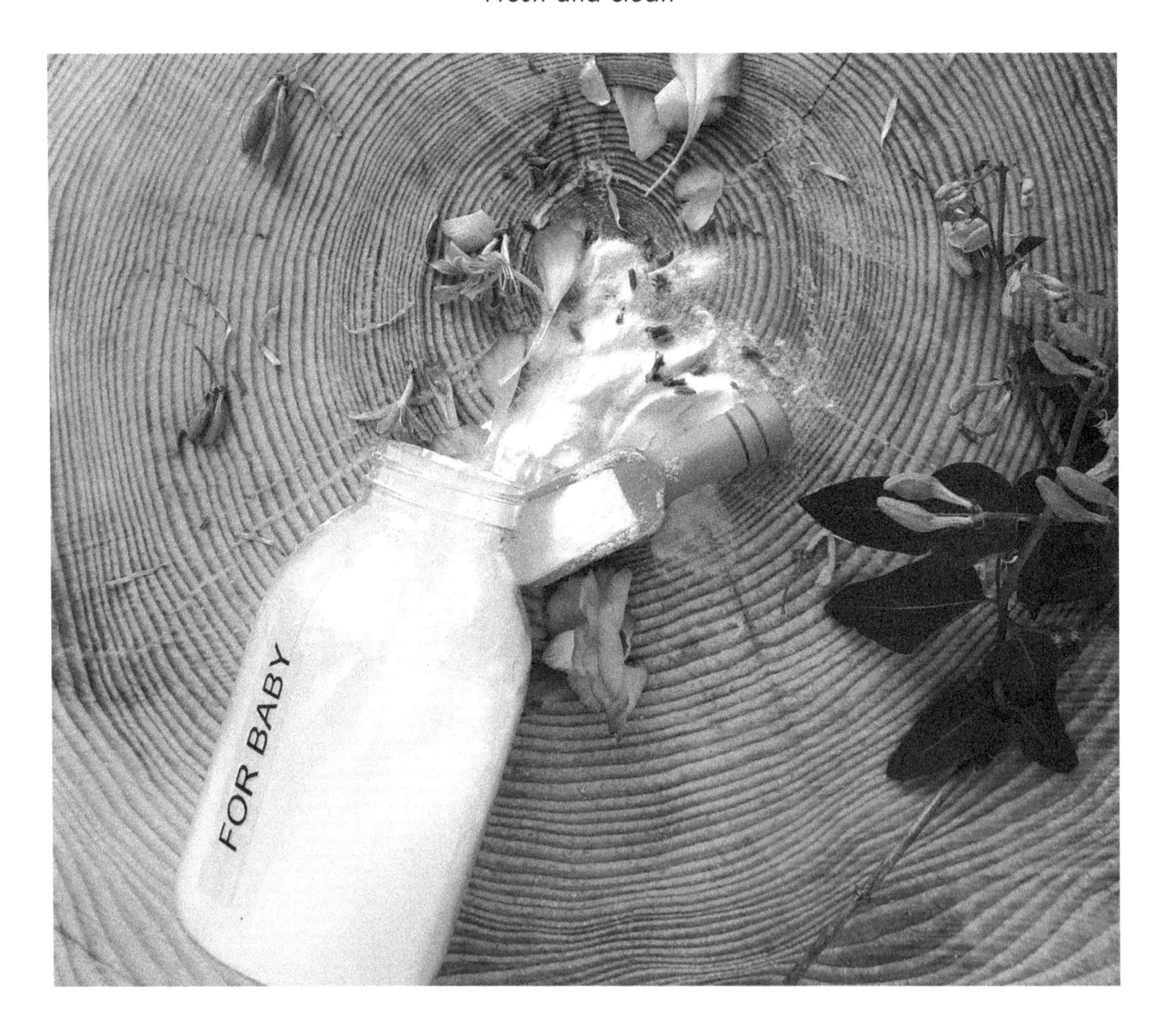

(Makes one 8oz jar)

Equipment list

- 8-oz mason jar with lid

Ingredients

- ¾ cup cornstarch
- ¾ cup arrowroot powder
- 1 TBSP baking soda

Instructions

1. Mix all dry ingredients together, and store in the mason jar.

Tips

You can easily double or triple the recipe if you want to make more.

Add lavender essential oil for a safe, pleasant scent.

Gentlest Baby Lotion

With no harmful ingredients

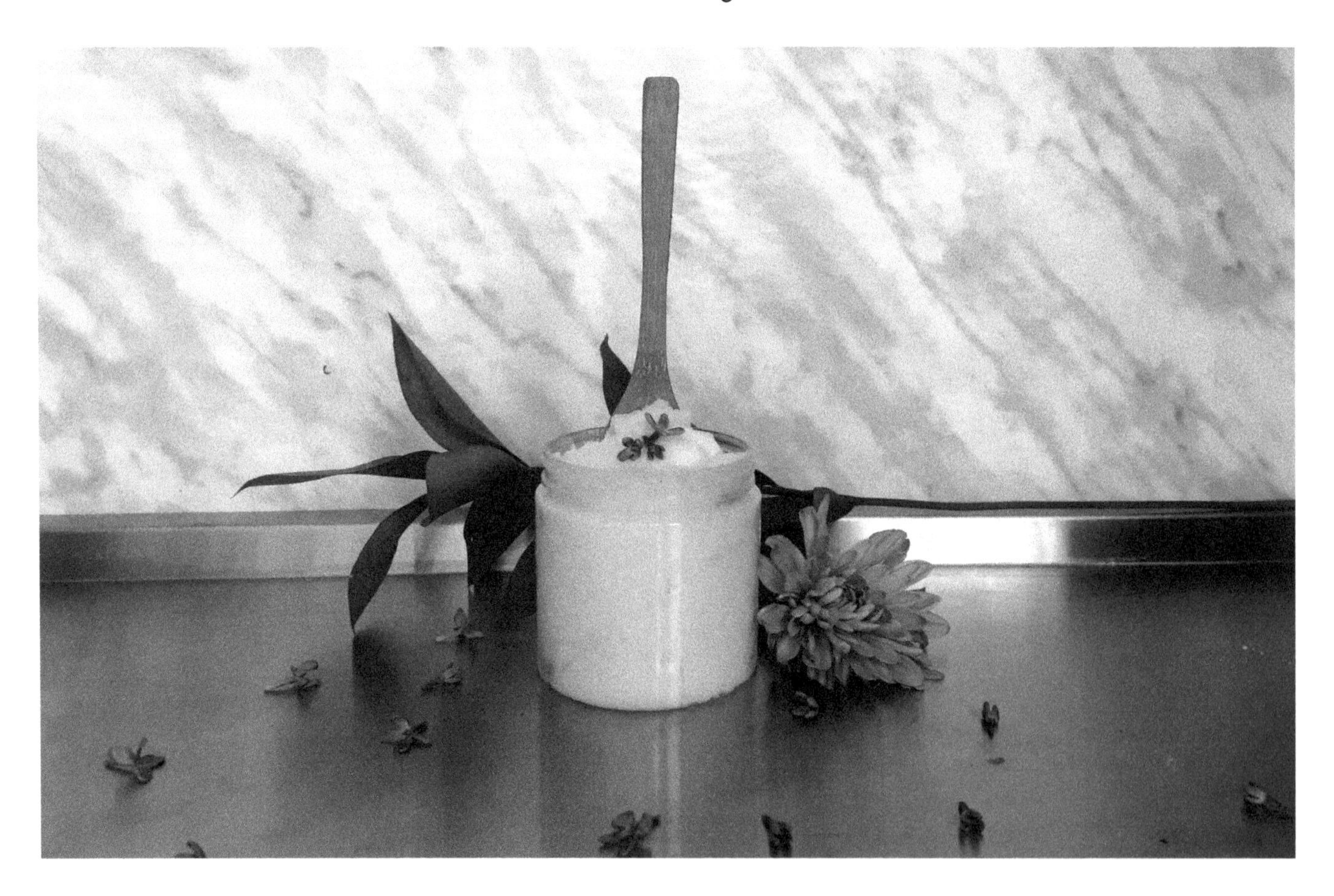

(Makes one 8 oz jar)

Equipment list

- 8-oz mason jar or glass container with lid
- Glass measuring cup

Ingredients

- ½ cup shea butter
- ½ cup organic coconut oil
- 2 TBSP beeswax
- 2 tsp vitamin E oil

Instructions

1. In a glass measuring cup, add the shea butter, coconut oil, and beeswax.
2. In the microwave, heat for 40 seconds. Stir, and return to the microwave for 30 seconds.
3. Continue stirring and heating for 30-second intervals until the mixture is liquid.
4. Add the vitamin E oil. Stir and pour into the container.

Tip

Allow to cool several hours or overnight.

Relaxing Baby Wash/Bath

After a busy day

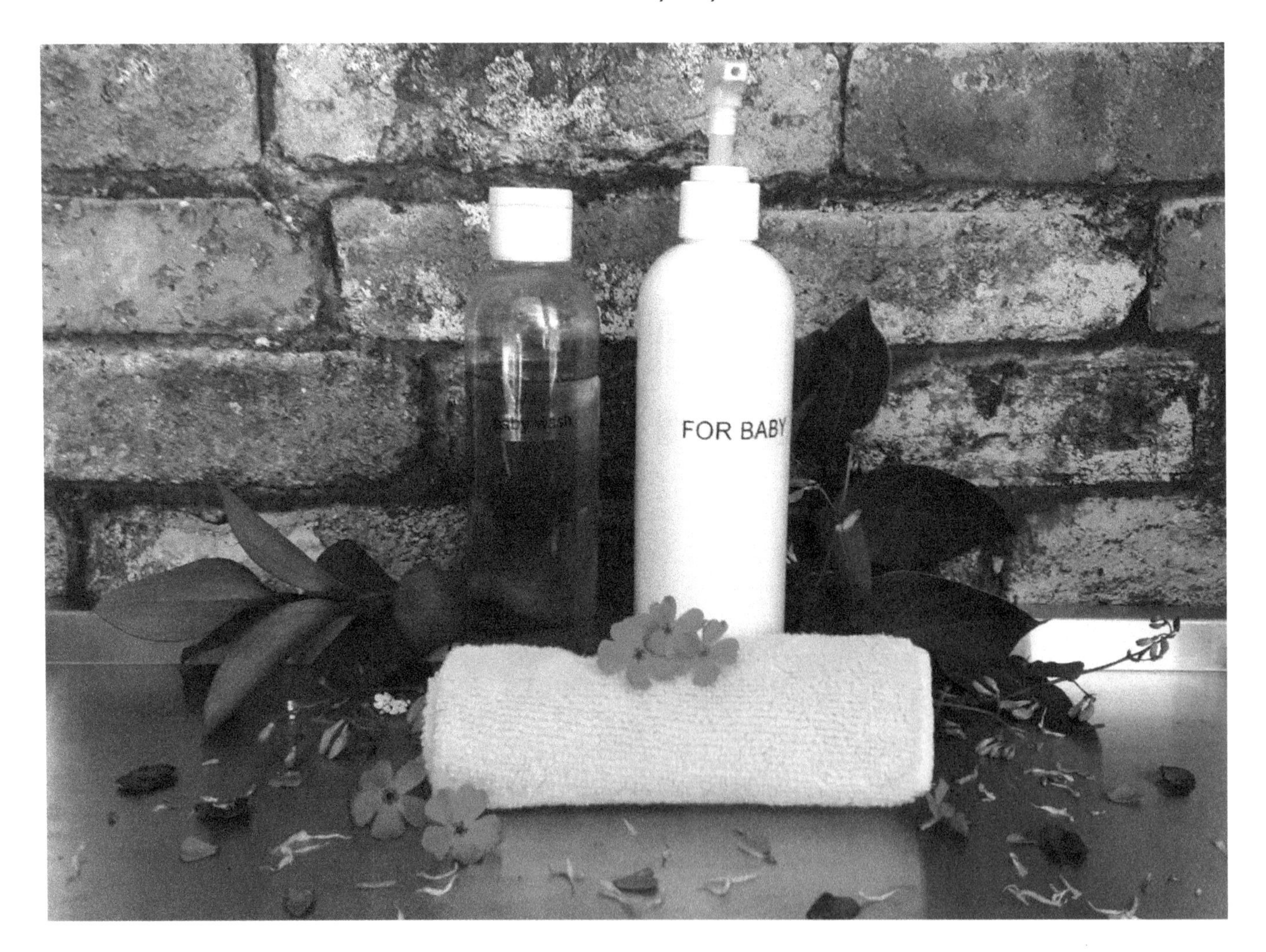

(Makes one 8 oz bottle)

Equipment list

- 8-oz container with a pump or dispenser
- 1 cup liquid castile soap (unscented)
- 2 TBSP plant-based glycerin
- 2 tsp coconut oil (liquid)
- 1 tsp vitamin E oil
- 2 TBSP water
- 3–10 drops lavender or chamomile essential oil

Ingredients

Instructions

1. Mix the above ingredients and place in a storage container.
2. You can add more water if you'd like a thinner solution. Perfect for bath time, and gentle on the skin.

Tip

We have recommended a very low, safe amount of essential oils for baby, or you can make it unscented.

THE AT-HOME SPA TREATMENT

Relax With Nature

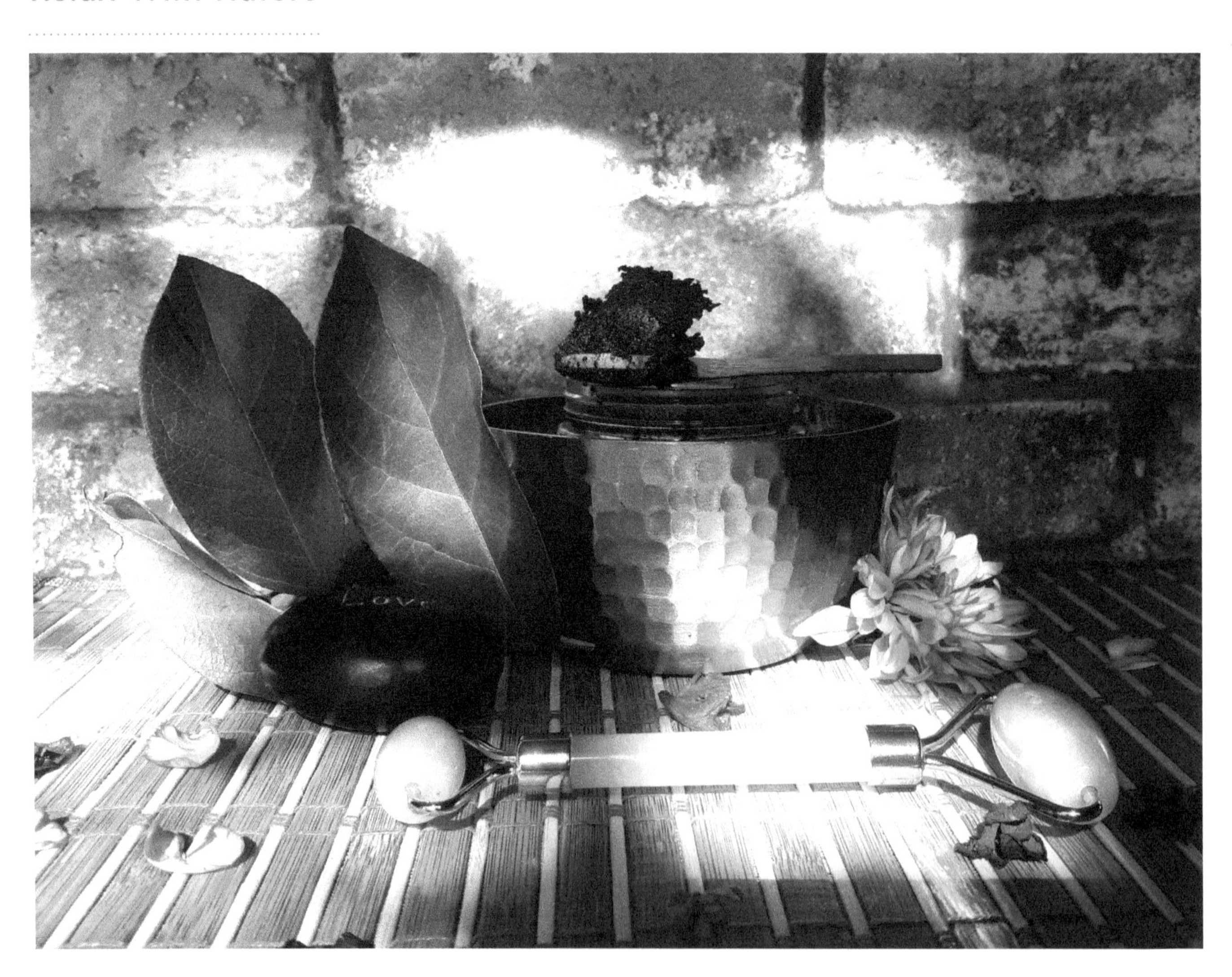

I love lazy Sundays with my daughter because that's a perfect day for a spa day. Here are my go-to spa treatments – think of all the money you'll save! Great recipes for your next ladies' night, cottage retreat, date night, and more!

You can make up the masks the day before if you prefer, or whip them up fresh. Either way, you are in for a relaxing treat!

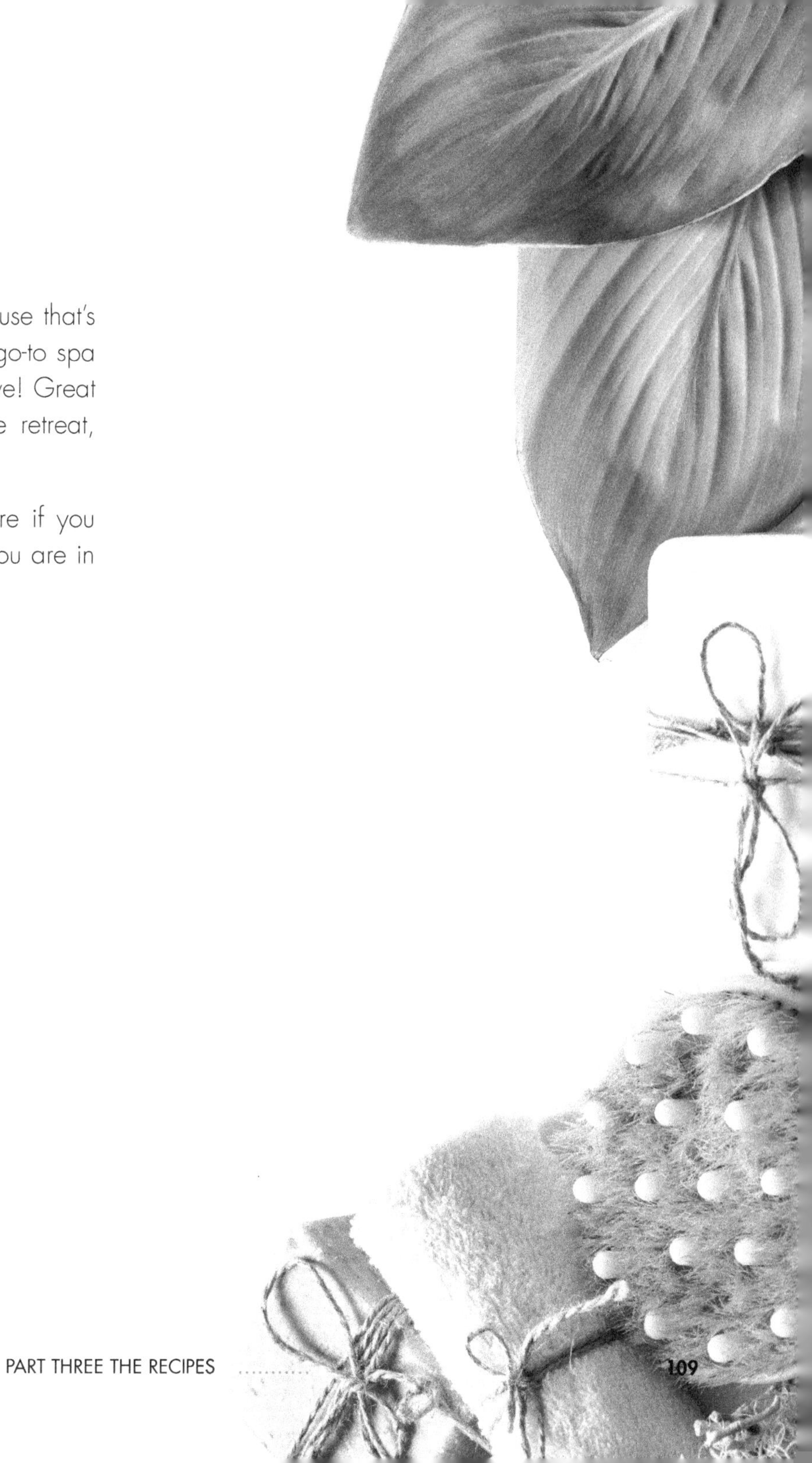

Glow-to Coffee Scrub and Mask

Good for aging and acne-prone skin

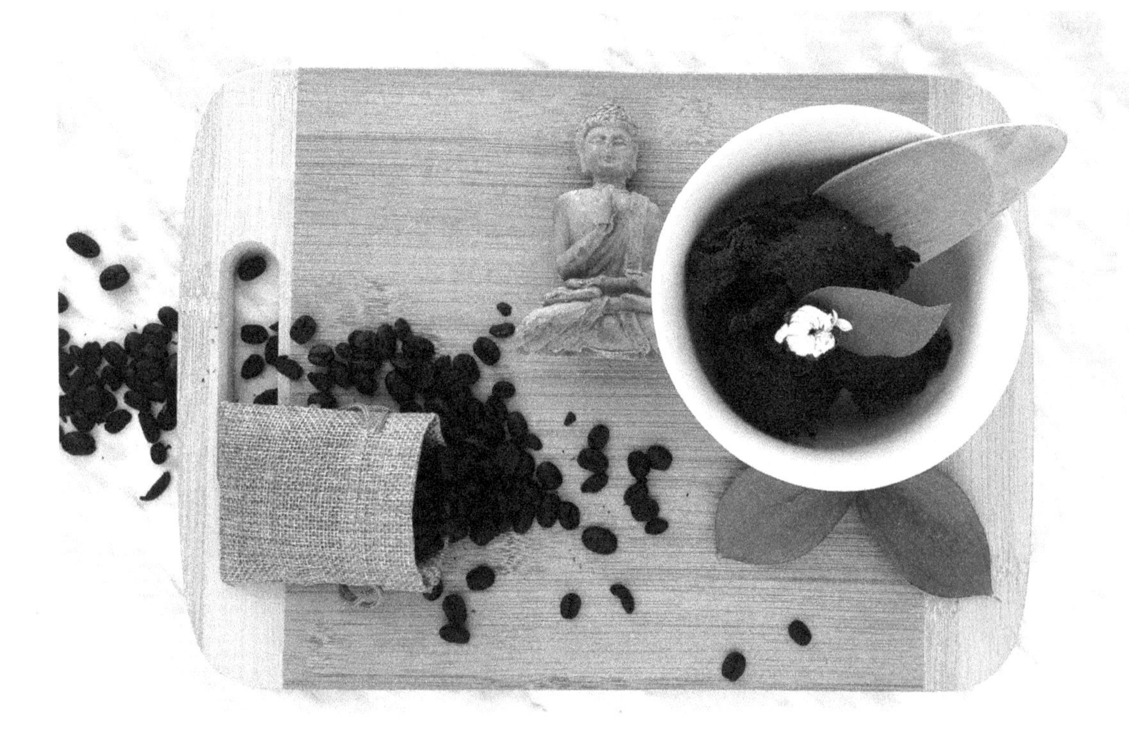

I love this all-purpose treatment. Make up a large batch and store in the fridge. This works great as an all-over body scrub to use in the shower, a foot scrub, and my fave facial mask.

Coffee is an amazing ingredient. For best results, use your leftover coffee grounds. The used grounds ensure the caffeine and coffee oils are released.

Coffee perks up the skin; it's an antioxidant and excellent for anti-aging and healing acne.

(Makes one 8 oz jar)

Equipment list

- 8-oz mason jar with lid
- Food processor

Ingredients

- 1 cup used coffee grounds or 1 cup fresh coffee grounds
- 1 cup organic coconut oil (semi-hard)
- 1 tsp vitamin E oil
- 30 drops tea tree oil

Instructions

1. In a food processor, mix the oil and the grounds
2. Once well-mixed, spoon into a clean, dry mason jar.
3. Store in the fridge.

Tips

Apply to your face or body daily or weekly. Rub in a circular motion.

You can leave it on your skin for 10 to 20 minutes. Rinse with warm water and pat dry.

You can store it in the fridge up to three months.

Peppermint Foot Scrub and Mask

Suitable for all skin types

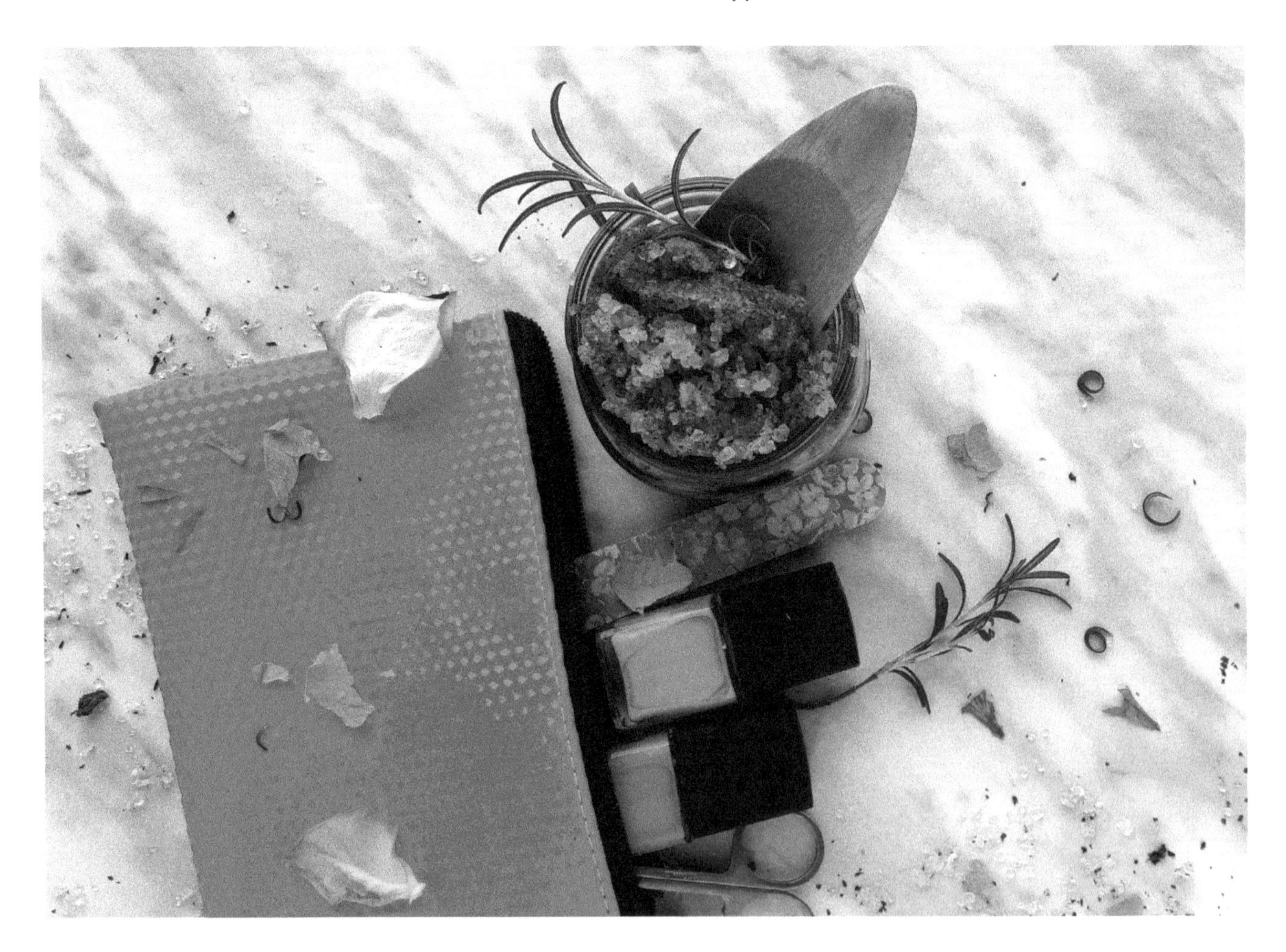

Add this to your pedicure regime. You will love how invigorating your feet feel afterward.

(Makes one 8 oz jar)

Equipment list

- 8-oz mason jar with lid
- Food processor

Ingredients

- 1 cup organic coconut oil (semi-hard)
- 1 cup cane sugar
- 1 tsp vitamin E oil
- 30 drops peppermint essential oil

Instructions

1. In a food processor, mix the oils and sugar.
2. Once mixture is smooth, spoon into a clean, dry container.

Tips

Apply daily or weekly.

Over a tub, towel, or basin, scrub your feet with about ¼ cup per foot.
It does get a little messy.

If you'd like to leave it on your feet longer as a foot mask,
wrap feet with plastic wrap or plastic bag. Leave on for 10 to 20 minutes.

Rinse with warm water and pat dry.

Deep Cleansing Detox Face Mask

Don't be afraid to get messy. All in the name of natural beauty!

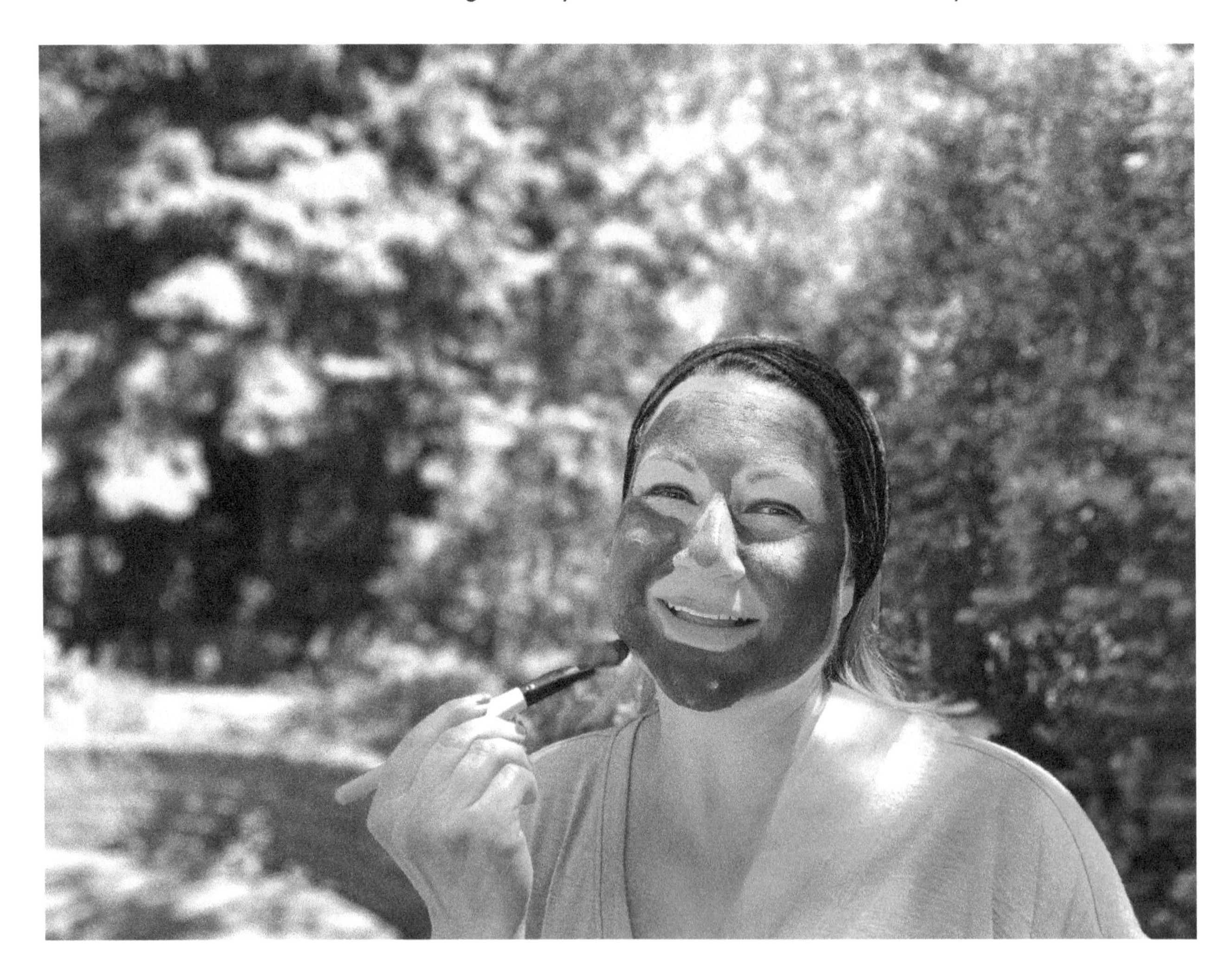

PHOTO CREDIT: **LAUREN BREWIN**

Activated charcoal is my go-to ingredient for detoxing.
It naturally removes toxins from the surface, which is really effective
when applying to the face. Dirt and oils will be washed away, leaving you with a clean face!

Equipment list

- Clean bowl to make the mask mixture
- Flat brush to apply the mask

Ingredients

- 1 TBSP activated charcoal
- 2 TBSP bentonite clay powder
- 1 TBSP fractionated coconut oil (liquid)
- 1 tsp apple cider vinegar
- 1 tsp water

Optional additions

- 10–15 drops rose or lavender essential oil

Instructions

1. Mix all ingredients together in a bowl until you have a thick paste. Add more water if needed.

Tips

Apply daily or weekly on a clean, dry face. Brush the mask on, avoiding eyes and mouth.

Leave on for 20 minutes or until dry and hard.

Gently remove with warm water and a dark wash cloth. Pat dry. Your face should feel firm and clean.

Matcha Green Face Mask

Chocked full of antioxidants

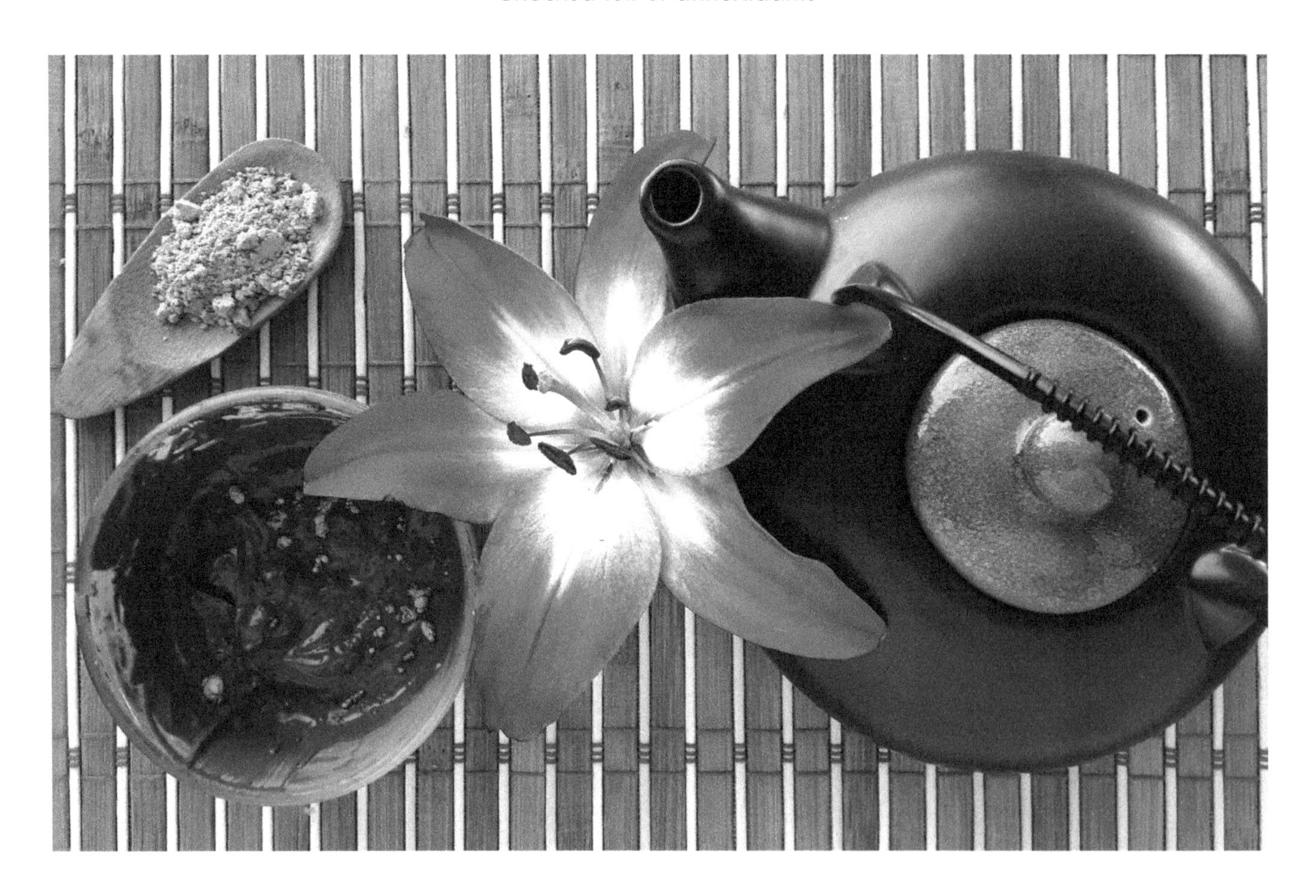

Great for anti-aging or acne. Has a beautiful green colour and earthy smell.
You can add essential oils if desired.

Equipment list

- Clean bowl to make the mask mixture
- Flat brush to apply the mask

Ingredients

- 2 TBSP matcha powder
- 2 TBSP bentonite clay powder
- 1 TBSP raw honey
- 1 tsp witch hazel
- 1 tsp water

Optional additions

- 10–15 drops chamomile or lavender essential oil

Instructions

1. Mix all ingredients together in a bowl until you have a thick paste.
2. Add more water if needed.

Tips

Apply daily or weekly on a clean, dry face; brush the mask on. Avoid eyes and mouth.

Leave on for 20 minutes or until dry and hard.

Gently remove with warm water and a wash cloth.

Pat dry. Your face should feel firm and clean.

Nourishing Hair Mask

Hydration for dry and damaged hair

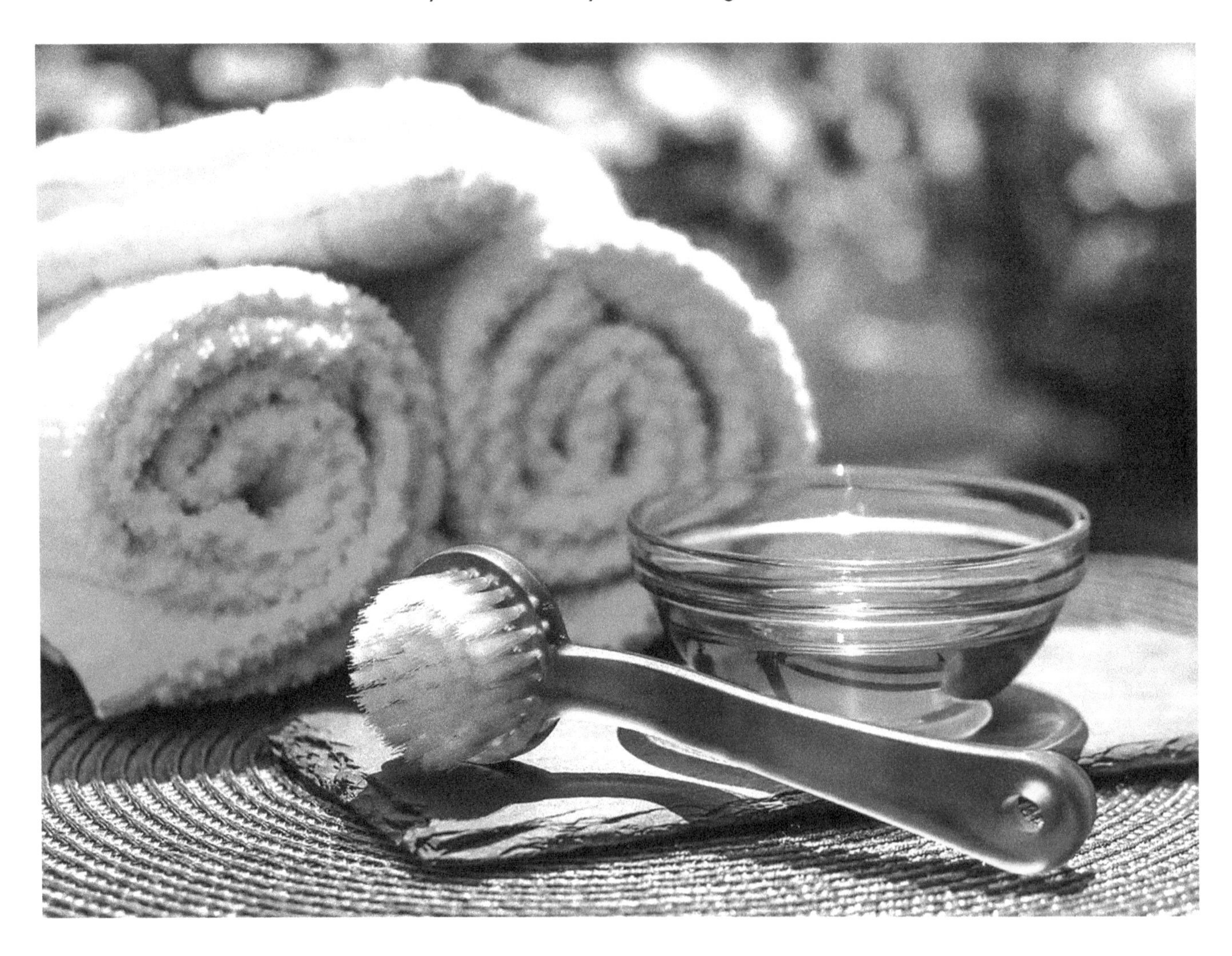

Equipment list

- Clean bowl to make the mask mixture
- Shower cap or plastic bag
- Towel

Ingredients

- ½ cup fractionated organic coconut oil (liquid)
- 2 TBSP liquid honey
- 1 tsp vitamin E oil
- 10 drops lavender essential oil

Instructions

1. Microwave the coconut oil and honey for about 30 seconds and stir until the honey is mixed well.
2. Add the vitamin E and essential oil.
3. Allow to cool for at least 10 minutes before applying to your hair.

Tips

Apply weekly. Over the tub, sink, or basin, cover your dry hair with the oil mixture.

Be sure to apply to your dry ends and avoid your scalp.

Cover your head with a shower cap or plastic bag, and then wrap with a warm towel.

Leave on for 20 to 30 minutes, and then rinse out.

Your hair will be shiny, not greasy, for days! You can do this mask once a week.

DIY GIFT-GIVING GUIDE

The Gift of Natural Healing

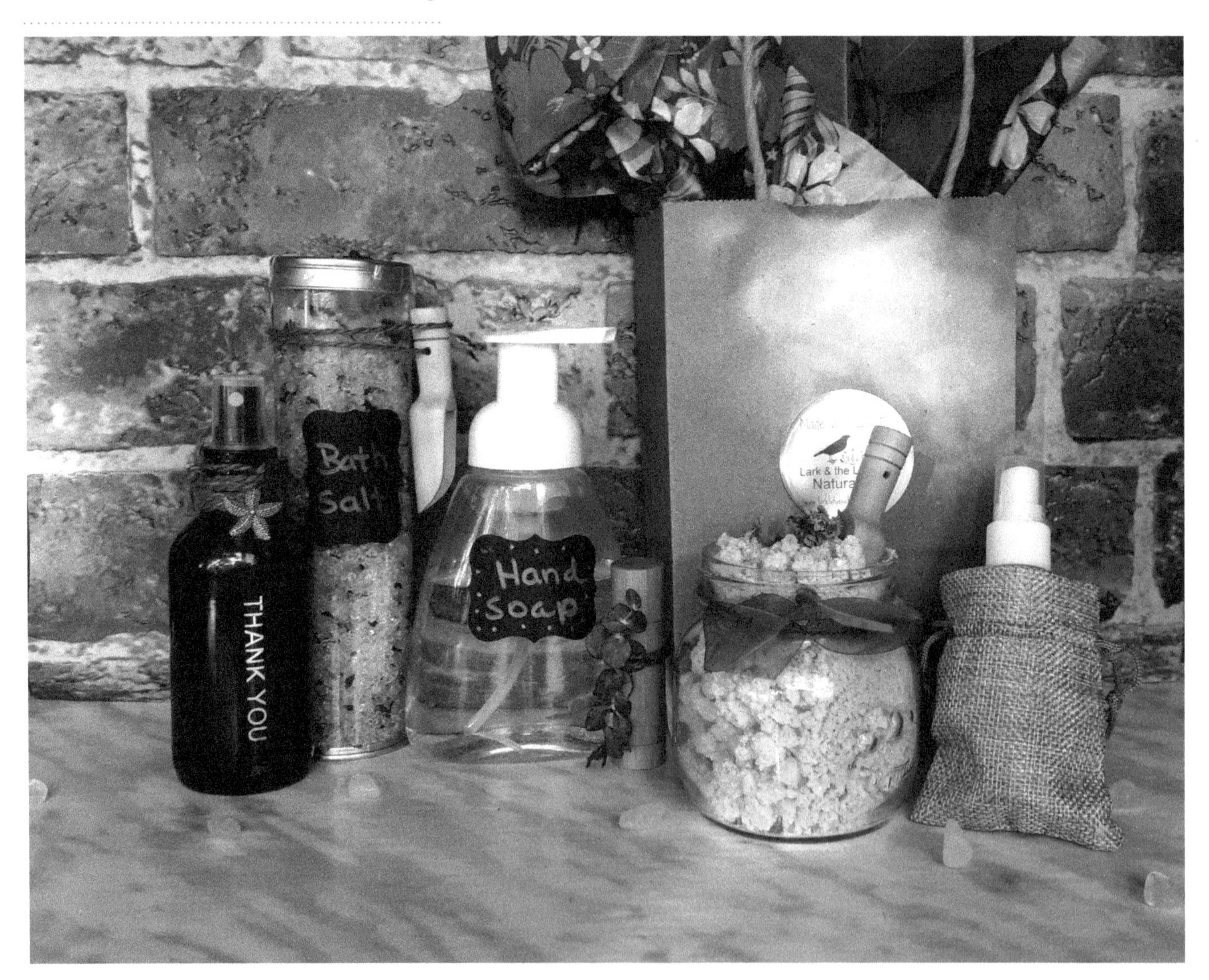

My favourite part of DIY is gift giving. I truly enjoy giving a personal gift I made myself to friends and family. DIY has come a long way and is now more popular than ever. People appreciate a handmade artisan gift. They look natural and appealing, and you can feel proud to put your name on it.

Here are some of my friends' and family's favourites to share with you!

For the teens

- Lip Scrub
- Lip Gloss

For the hostess

Invited to dinner? Bring one of these hostess gifts and you'll be in like flint!

- Hand Scrub
- Foaming Hand Wash

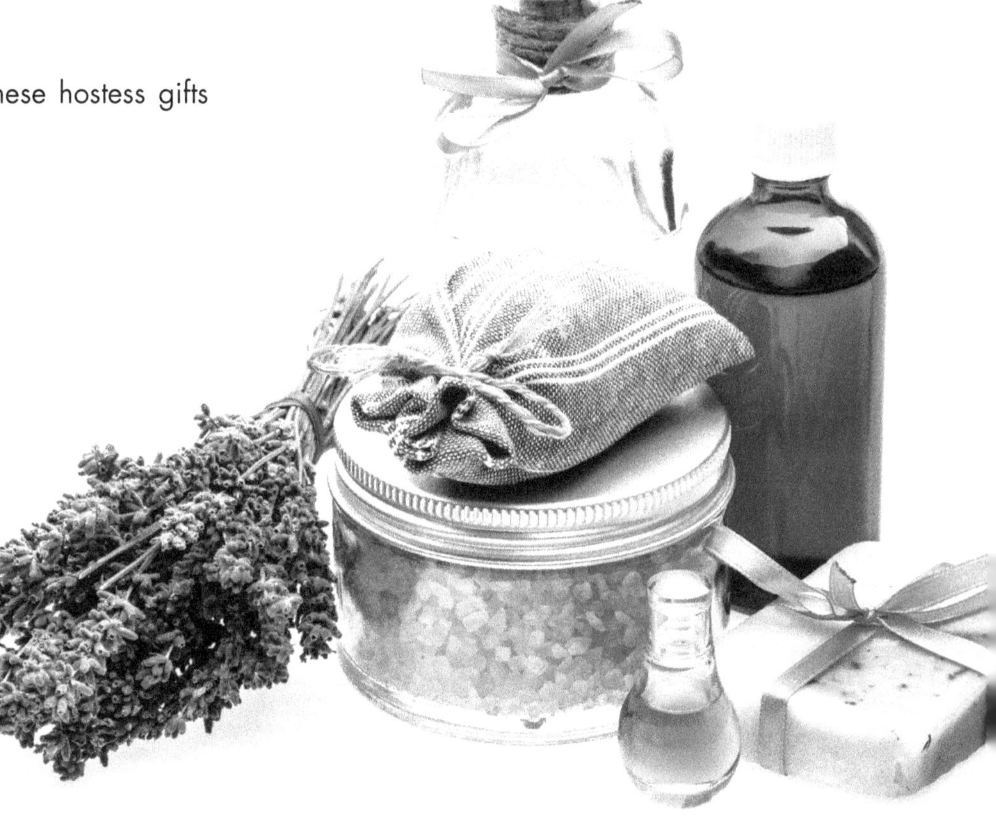

Lip Scrub Recipe

For soft, kissable lips

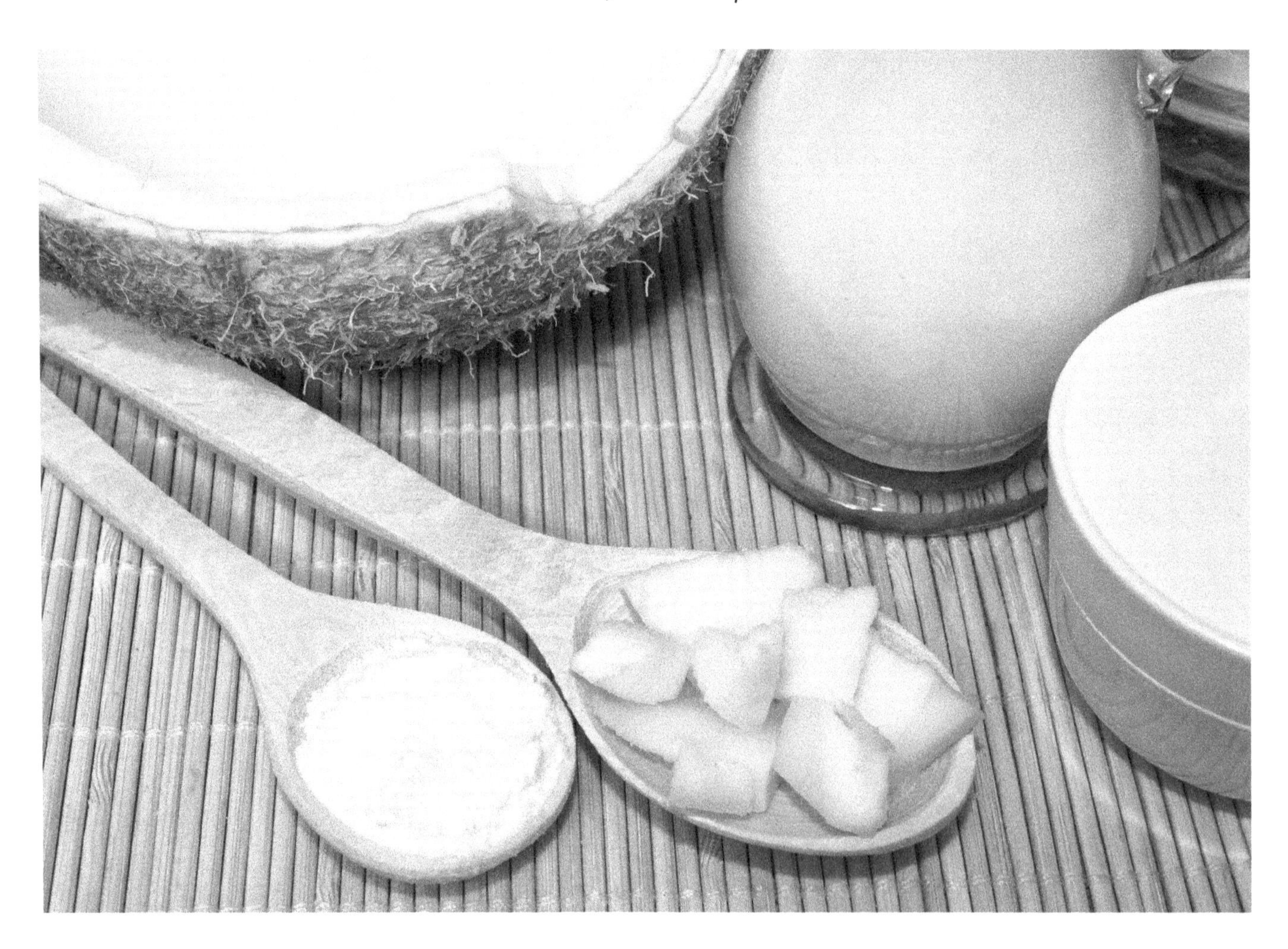

(Makes one small container)

Equipment list

- Small 4-oz container for your scrub

Ingredients

- ½ cup organic coconut oil (semi-hard)
- ½ cup raw cane sugar or brown sugar
- 10–20 drops essential oil of your choice

Instructions

1. In a bowl or food processor, mix the oil and sugar.
2. Add your essential oil of choice.

Tip

Store in a small container. Best used within three months.

Basic Lip Gloss

Add some drama to your pout

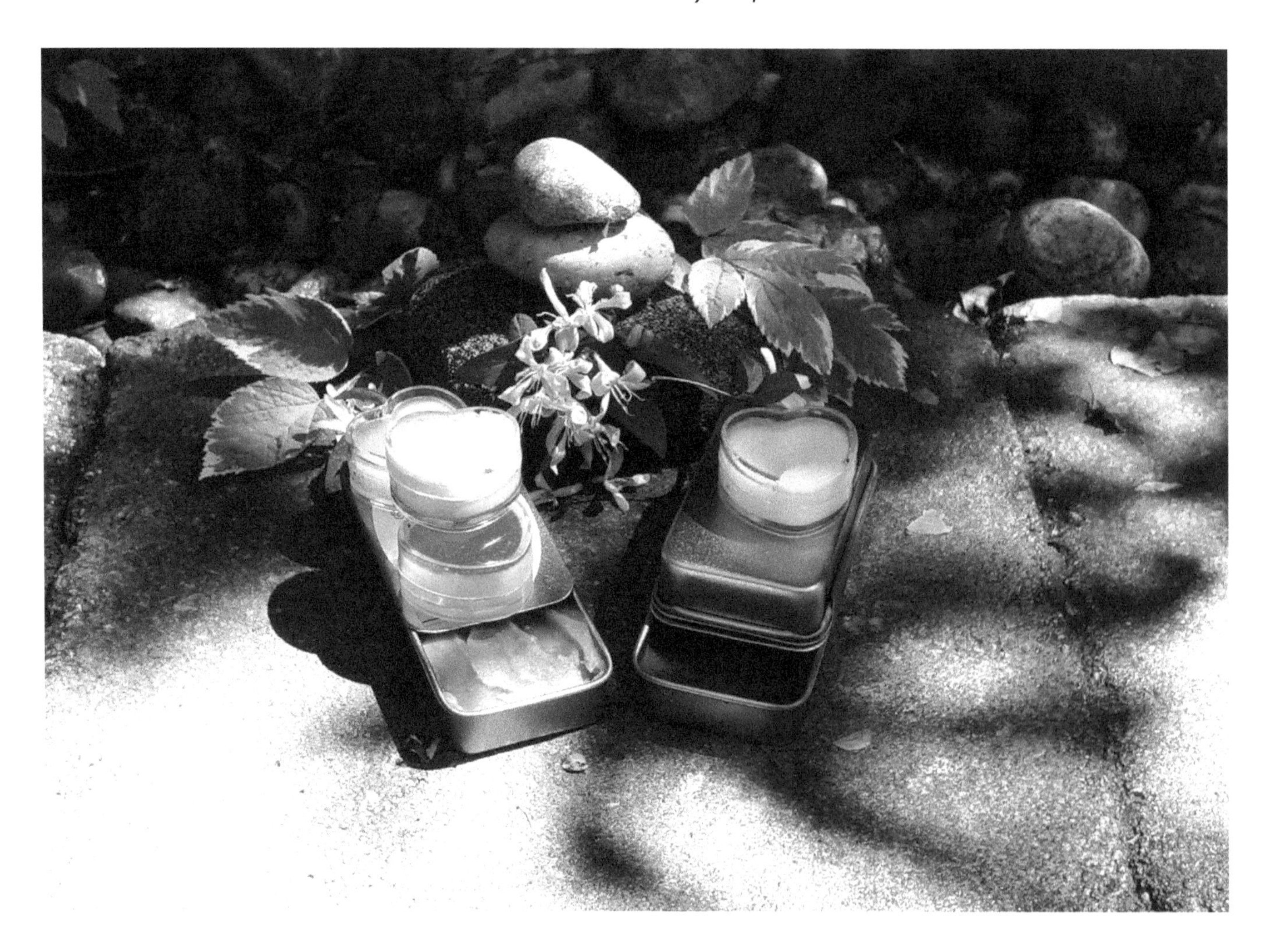

(Makes one small container)

Equipment list

- Small 2-oz container for your gloss

Ingredients

- 4 TBSP jojoba oil
- 1 TBSP beeswax
- 1 tsp honey
- ¼ tsp vitamin E oil
- 10 drops essential oil(s) of your choice

Optional additions

- 1 tsp hibiscus, beetroot, or cocoa powders for a natural tint

Instructions

1. Microwave the jojoba oil and beeswax in a glass measuring cup for 30 seconds.
2. Stir and repeat, heating for another 20 seconds or until mixture is melted.
3. Add vitamin E oil and your choice of essential oils.
4. To add a light colour to the gloss, use hibiscus, beetroot, or cocoa powder. The more you add, the deeper the tint.
5. Cool for 2 minutes, and then pour into a clean lip gloss container.
6. Chill for 1 hour in the fridge.

Tip

This gloss will be soft, so apply with a finger or makeup brush.

Lemon and Rosemary Hand Scrub

For soft and fresh-smelling hands

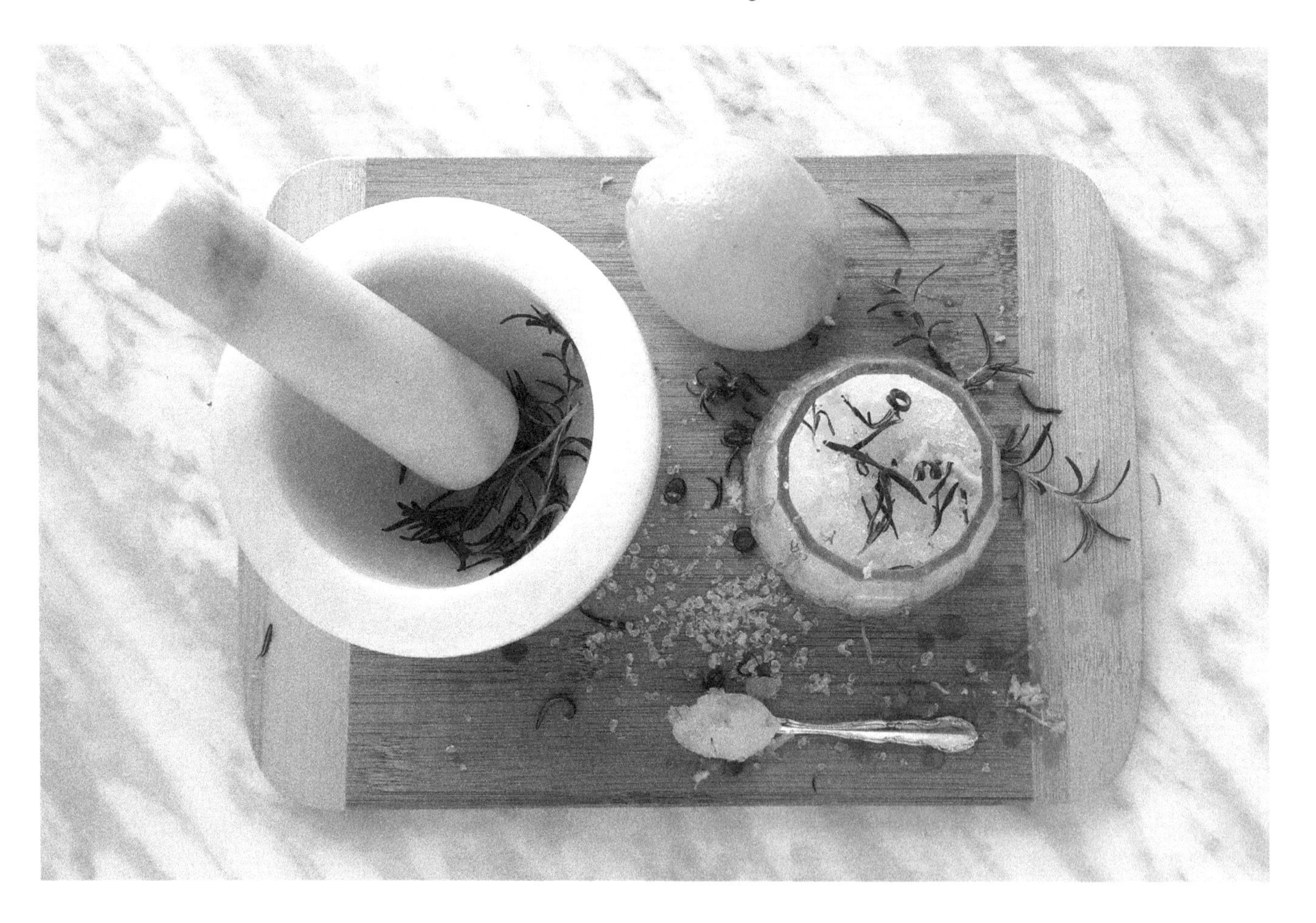

If you do your own cooking, you may agree that hands can smell like garlic and onions for days. This scrub will take that all away, leaving only a fresh smelling pair of hands and super baby-soft skin!

(Makes one small 6 oz container)

Equipment list

- 6-oz container with lid
- Food chopper or mortar and pestle
- Zester

Ingredients

- 1 organic lemon
- 3 TBSP fresh rosemary
- 1 cup coarse sea salt
- 3 TBSP olive oil

Instructions

1. Wash your lemon. Zest the peel. Set aside.
2. Juice the lemon.
3. In a mortar and pestle or food chopper, crush the rosemary into small bits approximately ½ cm in length.
4. In a clean bowl, mix the olive oil and salt.
5. Add 2 TBSP of lemon zest.
6. Add 2 to 3 TBSP of lemon juice.
7. Mix well, until the juice is absorbed. Spoon into a lovely container. And now you have a wonderful hostess gift.

Tip

Will last several months on the counter or in the fridge.

DIY Foaming Hand Wash

Easy and cost saving

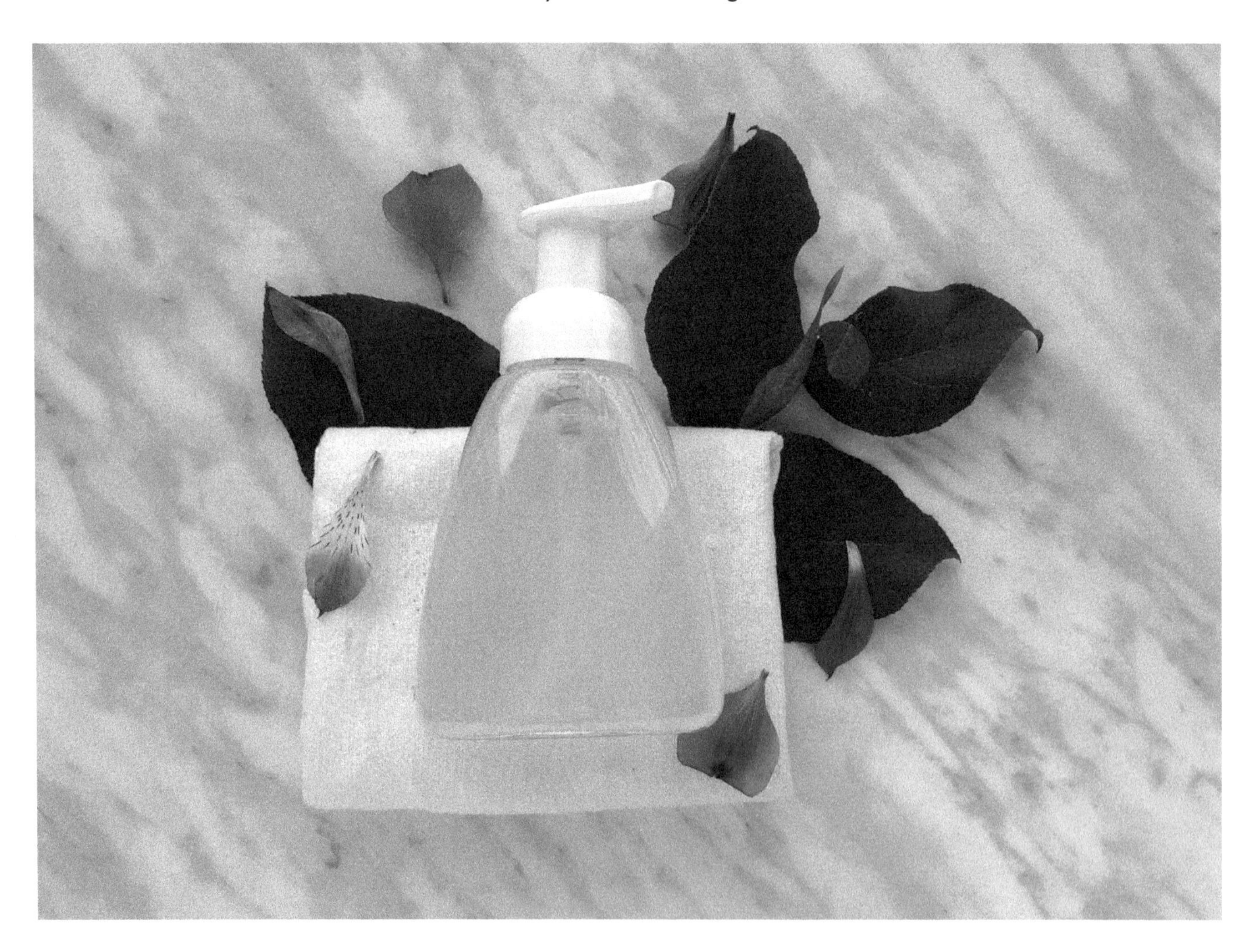

(Makes one 8 oz container)

Equipment list

- 8-oz foaming pump container

Ingredients

- ¼ cup liquid castile soap (unscented)
- 1 TBSP carrier oil of your choice
- 1 tsp of your favourite essential oil(s)
- Filtered or distilled water

Instructions

1. Mix the soap and carrier oil together. Add the essential oils.
2. In a clean pump bottle, pour the soapy mixture.
3. Fill the remainder of the bottle with clean filtered water, **leaving 1 inch** from the top.

Tips

It's important to leave at least a one-inch space at the top of the soap bottle so it can "foam."

Add a pretty label, and you have a great gift that will last months!

YOUR GREEN-CLEAN DAILY ROUTINE
Easy Steps to Take Each Day

I hope you've found this book helpful in eliminating chemicals from your daily routine. Most people don't miss their old products; in fact, they prefer the handmade versions of their favourites. It's nice to know exactly what's in each and every item you put on your body.

You can feel good about what you put in the shower for the family to use or what you use on your baby and young children. Plus, think of all the money you're saving!

Living clean is always a work in progress. Will we ever be 100% chemical free? Probably not, but every small change you make is making a big difference in your life and in others' lives.

Enjoy the feeling; you're worth the effort!

ACKNOWLEDGMENTS

This book would have remained a fleeting idea if it weren't for the following people:

My husband and children have been the driving force behind my desire to create a natural home environment. They have been especially patient and kind during this process, offering much support and interest in the project. So, thank you Michael, Lauren, and Ethan for your love and support.

I have been blessed with the most wonderful friendships. My girlfriends inspired me to launch my business, believed in me, and provided unconditional support and encouragement. Thank you Claire, Diana, Stephanie, and Wendy. I could not have done this without you.

To Sheri, thanks for all of your advice, ideas, and gentle pushes forward. Your mantra, "Do you have a book in you?" spoke to me during this journey and I am very thankful to have this opportunity to let the book out.

Special thanks to the staff and editors at Friesen Press.

Thank you to my sister Cathy, my nephew, and my niece for always boosting me up when I needed it, for listening to my ever-changing ideas, and for testing all the prototypes.

To all of my friends, colleagues, and customers in Barrie, Simcoe County, and my former hometown, Thunder Bay. Thank you for coming out to my shows, trying out products, and telling your friends and family about it. That is the best reward. Thank you!

For my mother, Connie. I dedicate this book to you. Thanks for giving me all the confidence I have and always making me feel unique, not different. I love you.

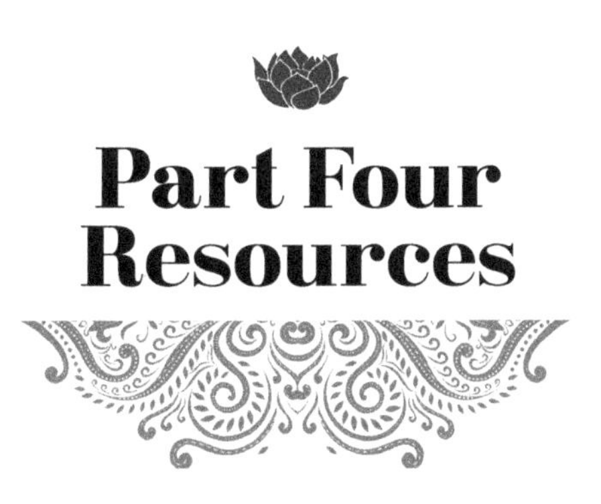

Part Four
Resources

MEASUREMENT CONVERSION TABLE

Teaspoons	Tablespoons	Ounces	Cups	Pints	Quarts	Gallons	Milliliters	Liters
3	1	1/2	1/16				15	0.015
12	4	2	1/4				60	0.06
24	8	4	1/2				125	0.125
48	16	8	1	1/2	1/4	1/16	250	0.25
		16	2	1	1/2	1/8	500	0.5
		32	4	2	1	1/4	950	0.95
		128	16	8	4	1	3800	3.8

WHERE TO SHOP

www.Amazon.ca or www.Amazon.com
For a variety of lip balm tubes and balls, raw materials, oils, beeswax, citric acid, carrier oils, essential oils.

Michaels Craft Store
For containers, beeswax, labels, ribbons, glass jars and containers.

www.Brambleberry.com
Fragrance oils and colorants.

The Dollar Store
Glass containers, labels, ribbons, embellishments, cake sprinkles.

Health Food Store
Natural colourants, teas, dried flowers, organic raw materials, baking soda, cornstarch, extracts, carrier oils, essential oils.

END NOTES

1 Yao-Ping Lu *et al*, "Tumorigenic Effect of Some Commonly Used Moisturizing Creams when Applied Topically to UVB-Pretreated High-Risk Mice," National Center for Biotechnology Information, published online August 14, 2008. ncbi.nlm.nih.gov/pmc/articles/PMC2630214/?tool=pubmed

2 C.M. Vrabie *et al*, "Specific in vitro toxicity of crude and refined petroleum products: II. Estrogen (alpha and beta) and androgen receptor-mediated responses in yeast assays," NCBI, 2011. ncbi.nlm.nih.gov/pubmed/20821602

SOURCES

Campaign for Safe Cosmetics. A project of Breast Cancer Prevention Partners, which works to protect the health of consumers, workers, and the environment. safecosmetics.org

Concin, N., Hofstetter, G., Plattner, B., Tomovski, C., Fiselier, K., Gerritzen, K., Semsroth, S., *et al.* "Evidence for cosmetics as a source of mineral oil contamination in women." NCBI. October 4, 2001. ncbi.nlm.nih.gov/pubmed/21970597

Useful information

Campaign for Safe Cosmetics. A campaign that uses smarts and sass to pressure the cosmetics industry to make safer products. Educates about the problem of toxic chemicals in cosmetics, which has led to increased demand for safer products by both the public and retailers. safecosmetics.org

Environmental Working Group. An online guide with safety ratings for more than 78,000 cosmetics and other personal care products and more than 25,000 brands. ewg.org/skindeep/site/about.php

People for the Ethical Treatment of Animals: Beauty Without Bunnies. A searchable database of companies that do and do not test their products on animals. peta.org/living/beauty-and-personal-care/companies/default.aspx

Photo credits

Photos of Susan courtesy of Nat Caron Photography
Lifestyle Photos courtesy of Susan Brewin
Pixabay Free Stock Images

ABOUT THE AUTHOR

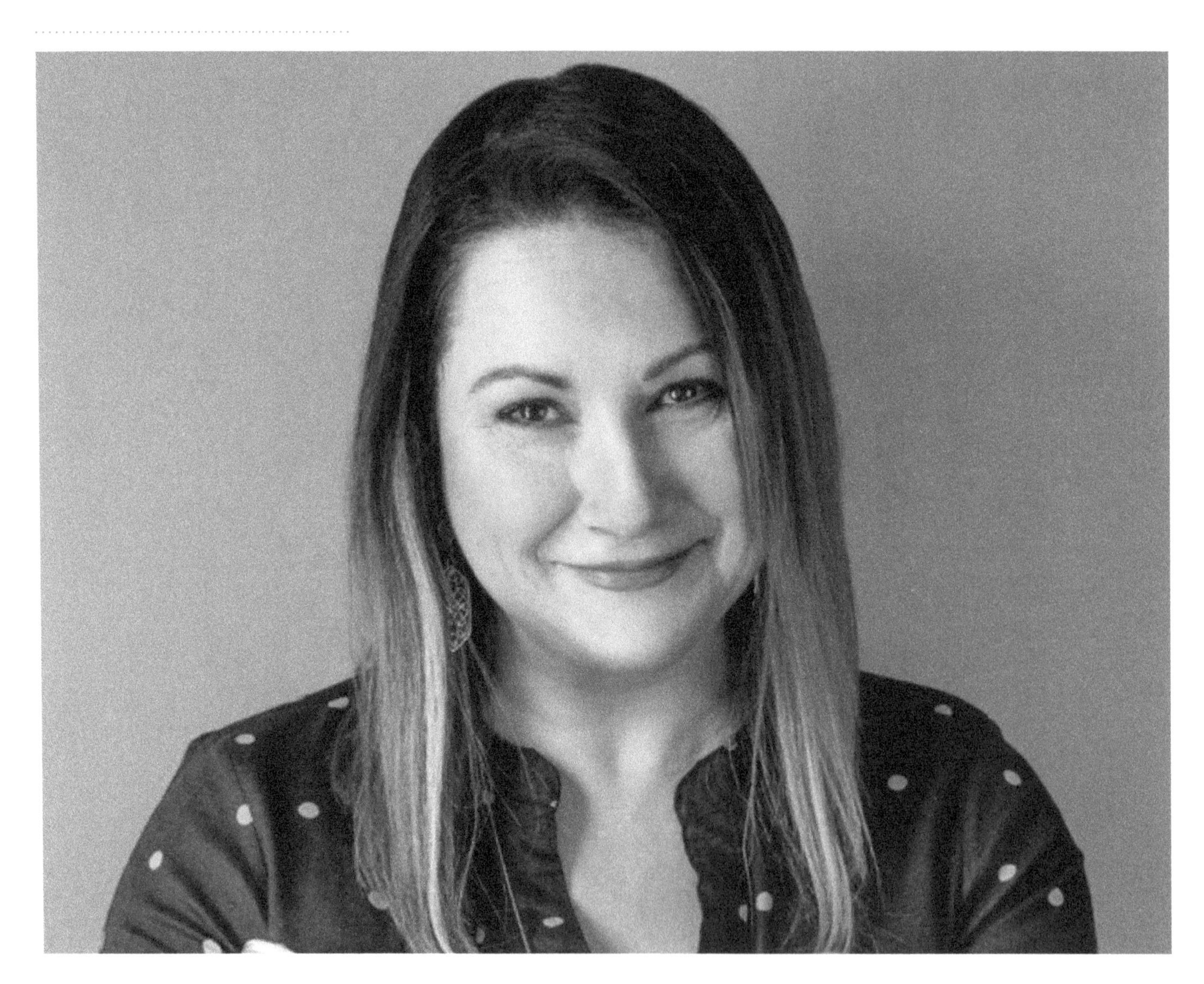

SUSAN BREWIN is passionate about health and wellness. She is a certified Aromatherapist, Crystal Healer, Reiki Practitioner, and Photographer. She currently resides in Southern Ontario, Canada.

As a conscientious mom and entrepreneur, Susan decided to take control of the personal-care products the family was using each day on their bodies, and in their home. Disappointed to learn that the expensive, so-called "natural" products contained harmful chemicals and fragrances that can cause long-term illness, hormone imbalance, cancer, allergies and more.

Susan became determined to find a solution for her family and quickly realized the most trust-worthy products are made at home. She began creating a full line of natural personal-care products for the whole family.

Susan is excited to share her favourite product recipes with you.

To learn more about, or purchase Susan's natural products visit www.larklotusnaturals.com

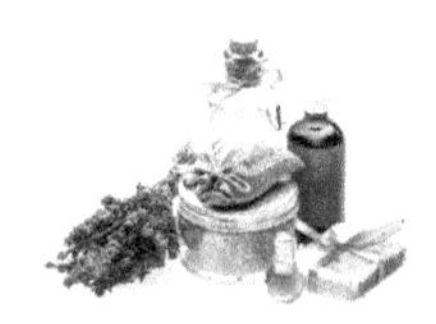
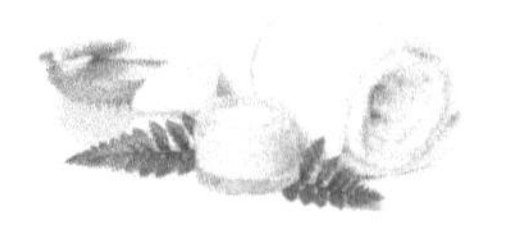
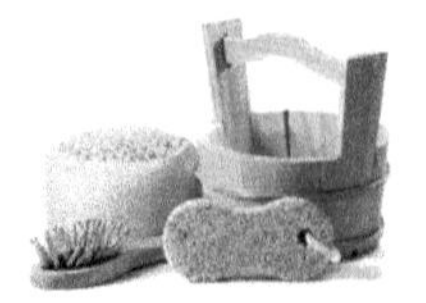

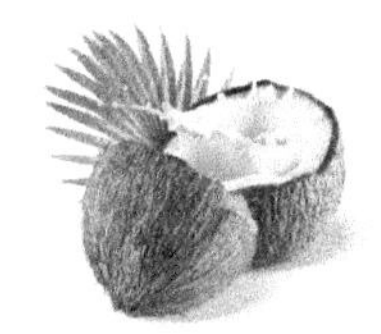
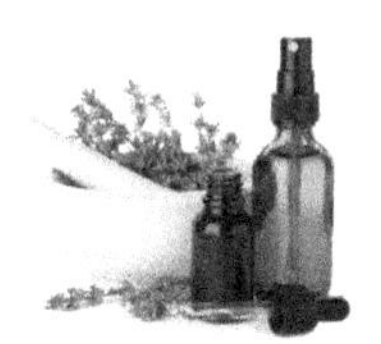
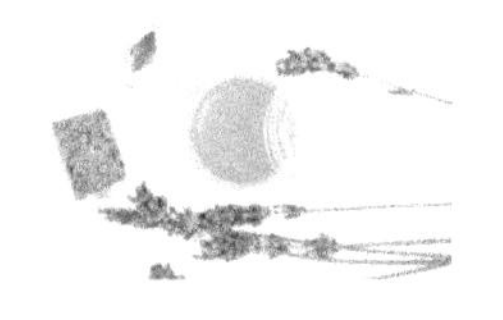
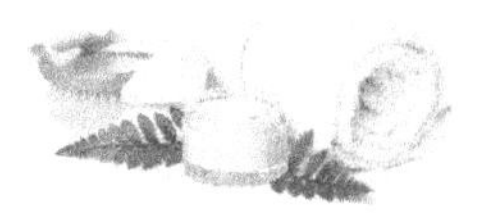

CPSIA information can be obtained
at www.ICGtesting.com
Printed in the USA
LVHW071634120420
653019LV00002B/4